The Gym Life Essays

Improve Your Life Through Fitness, Food, and Mindset

By Colin Stuckert
www.aGymLife.com

Disclaimer:

ISBN: 0615892426
ISBN 13: 9780615892429
LCCN Imprint Name: GymLife

Welcome to The Gym Life

My name is Colin Stuckert and I want <u>You</u> to live a better life. It sounds simple but it is definitely the most difficult thing in the world to get <u>You</u> to do. <u>You</u> love your habits, <u>You</u> love seeking comfort and avoiding pain, <u>You</u> love to chase externals, <u>You</u> avoid introspection, and <u>You</u> don't want to challenge your ego. Worst of all, <u>You</u> prefer comfort and maintaining the status quo. With all things in life worth having, change comes beyond all of these things that <u>You</u> like to do. Change comes past the burn, as Arnold would say. It comes past comfort; in fact, it most often comes only through pain and suffering.

A little about me before we get back to <u>You</u>. In 2009 I founded The Training Box—a group fitness and MMA gym—in sunny Southwest Florida. I have been learning, coaching, and helping people get better on a daily basis since then. It's been an amazing journey with plenty of ups and downs. I've experienced success and failure—professionally and personally—along the way. A sad statistic is I've seen more clients fail than succeed in pursuing their fitness goals. In fact, the percentage of clients that stick with it for the long run is probably in the single digits. Trust me, it is that bad. I've seen hundreds of motivated and perfectly capable people program hop, yo-yo, quit completely, and give every excuse in the book as to why they can't keep going. This disgusting prevalence of failure I've encountered over the years has motivated me to write. My goal with the book you hold in your hands is to help <u>You</u> avoid becoming just another one of these statistics.

My life right now looks like this: I run two businesses, write for my blog (agymlife.com), mentor, travel, manage employees, train, cook most of my meals from scratch, learn new skills when motivated, watch movies, read books, and study philosophy, psychology, and business. It seems like quite a bit from the outside looking in, but I actually have a lot of free time (lately anyways). This is because I've invested heavily in my personal knowledge and habits over the years. I've found that the more you understand about your body and mind, the easier it is to set and reach goals (which is a low probability occurrence for most people).

When you have better control over your thoughts, you will have better control over making decisions that will result in progress towards your goals. The more often you make these *good* decisions, the more likely you will form them into habits. Then, once these habits are formed, it's cakewalk. Ultimately, this is where success comes from: Your habits. A goal is simply an expression of a million action steps performed through habit. And once you form these habits, your goals will become a simple expression of time; it will become *not if, but when.*

Now for the bad news: <u>The majority of you reading this will never reach the body and health you want and deserve</u>. You won't invest the time, make the sacrifices, and stay the course long enough to get there. This totally sucks, and I wish it wasn't the case, but we must face the facts.

My Mission

My mission is to save as many people as I can by arming them with the proper knowledge and mindset. I'm hoping you will be one of them. By now you probably have one of two thoughts. The large percentage of you will scoff, ignore my warnings, and continue living your life full of denial. The rest—a much smaller percentage—will be encouraged. It will light a fire under your ass and you will be forced into action. Something will click in your head and you will start the process. Hopefully, since you purchased this book, you will be this minority percent and it will be a calling to you. If you are in the other group, and you prefer to live in a blanket of denial, than I suggest you follow these steps:

> 1. Send me an email with the following subject: The introduction offended me because I can't handle the truth
>
> 2. Include in the body: Please refund my purchase price via PayPal (include PayPal email address)
>
> 3. Give the book to someone else that will benefit from it

While this might seem a bit depressing, you must realize that I'm just being honest with you. We must face the facts, even if they aren't pleasant. You can't escape the human condition. Your mindset is going to keep you fat, sick, depressed, and not reaching your goals. Or your mindset is going to provide you longevity, a body you love, and worldly success for the rest of your life. It all comes down to the root: You. Notice all the You's underlined. This is to iterate that the only person in this equation is You. No one can do it for you. You make the choice or not and that's all there is to it.

The formula of fitness and health is simple to understand yet everyone loves to complicate it. Instead of obsessing over trying to find the 'perfect' system, focus on the basics:

Skip the junk food, sleep a lot, exercise a few times a week, believe in something, spend time with friends and family, get outdoors, and don't cry over spilt milk (don't stress yourself).

Simple right? Of course it's simple, but it's also wildly difficult (at first, at least). It can take months, even years, to build the habits necessary to sustain a high level of adherence to a healthy lifestyle. It can be very hard, to say the least. But does that mean we make excuses? Hell no. It means we work that much harder now that we understand what it's going to take.

A word you will see often in the following text is *nonnegotiable*. I use this word often because certain concepts for health and fitness are 100% nonnegotiable. You cannot skimp, skip, or ignore something that is nonnegotiable (like sleep, for example). This word also applies in an overall sense to everything in your life. Your body, mind, and health are the only things you actually posses in this world and no amount of money, success, or accomplishment will ever give you back the damage you do to yourself by forgoing the principles of health. *Your health is nonnegotiable.* You can't sacrifice any aspect of it and not pay the price of consequence. It's time to stop messing around with drugs, shitty food, all-nighters, and telling yourself that you will 'start' tomorrow. Time to put an end to excuses and cop-outs. Every decision you make is a chance to improve your health.

It's time to get working and develop the habits that will keep you healthy the rest of your life.

My urge here is to go off on a rant about the food industry, drugs, our fat-sick country, daughters losing their mothers to breast cancer, sons losing their fathers to heart disease, young people getting cancer and disease at record low ages, childhood obesity (abuse), impotence, survival of the fittest, the weak and pathetic modern man, conspiracy theories, the government, and how all of this is like global warming—an inconvenient truth—but I will spare you, for now.

The Bottom Line is if you don't have the physical body you want, you have no one to blame but yourself; only you have the power.

How your body looks and feels is 100% within your doing, for better or worse. If you don't have the body you want and need someone to blame, blame yourself. Actually, scratch that. Blaming yourself isn't going to make you feel any better, so drop that negative self-talk, drop the blame game, and start the start game. The start game involves you getting off your ass and dropping that negative-excuse-ridden-weak-mindset. For the gym warriors thinking that this text doesn't apply to you, I want you to think long and hard about what you do at the expense of your health. I guarantee that you need improvement somewhere, just like the rest of us. We all have our weaknesses. Maybe for you it's a crappy diet, lack of sleep, or too much booze? This is a calling for you to get better regardless of where you are in the process (and regardless of how good you look standing in front of a mirror).

Excuses are just a figment of your imagination created by your brain to avoid pain. Excuses are created in the mind to keep you on the path of least resistance. The best way to crush these excuses is to simplify the equation. Educate yourself. Remind yourself that there is a destination and a path to get there. That's all that matters. You decide that you will do the work necessary or not. That's it.

RESISTANCE in all caps

I want you to stop reading, right now, and do 30 push-ups. Don't put it off until later and don't brush it off as pointless. Quiet those excuses that are undoubtedly running through your head. This friction in your mind is called "Resistance" and it has manifested itself to keep you from doing the work. <u>And this is exactly what I want you to take notice of</u>. Your initial thoughts were probably, "ya right" or "later" or "I get the point so I don't need to actually do the push-ups." Well, you need to wage World War 3 on that BS. This aversion to doing is what David Pressfield calls Resistance in "The War of Art." Resistance is why you aren't where you want to be in every aspect of your life and it's goes well beyond doing a few push-ups. Listen up:

From The War of Art by David Pressfield (Trust me, buy this book now.):

Resistance is fear. But Resistance is too cunning to show itself naked in this form. Why? Because if Resistance lets us see clearly that our own fear is preventing us from doing our work, we may feel shame at this. And shame may drive us to act in the face of fear.

Resistance doesn't want us to do this. So it brings in Rationalization. Rationalization is Resistance's spin-doctor. It's Resistance's way of hiding the Big Stick behind its back. Instead of showing us our fear (which might shame us and impel us to do our work), Resistance presents us with a series of plausible, rational justifications for why we shouldn't do our work.

What's particularly insidious about the rationalizations that Resistance presents to us is that a lot of them are true. They're legitimate. Our wife may really be in her eighth month of pregnancy; she may in truth need us at home. Our department may really be instituting a changeover that will eat up hours of our time. Indeed it may make sense to put off finishing our dissertation, at least till after the baby's born.

What Resistance leaves out, of course, is that all this means diddly. Tolstoy had thirteen kids and wrote War and Peace. Lance

Armstrong had cancer and won the Tour de France three years and counting.

Pressfield, Steven (2011-11-11). The War of Art (pp. 55-56). Black Irish Entertainment LLC. Kindle Edition.

This aversion-based mindset is why you don't have what you want in life (remember it's only up to you). It is our human nature to make reasons to say no, to make excuses and stay in our bubble of comfort. The successful get working and get their hands dirty. This is the only way to get there--through hard work and constant action. Try to find reasons to say yes in your life. Life gets lived by people that say yes. Fit people are "yes" people. Find reasons to say yes to yourself. Your relationships, work, fitness, and health will improve. I guarantee it.

Did you actually do those push-ups? If so, you will get it done and it's going to be awesome. Just stay the course and you will get there. For you though, I have slightly different advice: *prepare yourself for success*. Remind yourself that you deserve success and be ready to accept it. As ridiculous as that sounds, many sabotage their results because they are scared of success. They have deep-seeded limiting beliefs that subconsciously tell themselves that they don't deserve success. The closer you get to success, the more you can find ways to screw it up and do dumb shit. This is a serious matter ladies and gentlemen. These limiting beliefs are lying in the weeds and most have no idea they are there. You must welcome success, embrace it, and remind yourself that you do deserve it.

Remember, life is brutally short and we are all just specks of sand in the grand scheme of the universe. If you want to make your life the best it can be during the infinitesimal amount of time you have, than you will have to utilize every second of every day to live the best you can. If you can make this your daily habit—to live fully—you will create an amazing life for yourself.

My Name is Colin Stuckert and I Believe in Fitness

We all face struggles in life. Some people have excellent genetics, become professional athletes, and seem to have it made. So what? Maybe they aren't happy? Maybe they never find true love? Maybe they suffer tragedy and loss? Maybe they die young? **Don't judge or compare.** Comparing is the perfect way for your mind to make excuses. Worrying about what others are doing, and making assumptions based on this, is a losing proposition. Slipping into the comparison trap is dangerous for your results. Your brain is always looking for the path of least resistance and you must be vigilant in not giving it any reasons to do so.

Some of us are celiac while others are less sensitive to gluten. Some can eat massive amounts of junk food and not gain a pound while others seem to gain weight on a clean diet. As we consider nutrition and exercise and how they are analogous to medicine, you will see that our bodies are governed by a few universal rules. Within these rules there are hundreds, if not thousands, of permutations. This is why self-testing is so important. You must find the perfect formula for yourself. The foundation looks something like this:

- •Natural diet consisting of healthy animals and plants

- •Resistance training (weightlifting)

- •Brief periods of high-intensity conditioning (sprinting, interval training)

- •Lots of walking/moving at a slow-to-medium pace

- •Proper lifestyle (sleep, sunlight, stress management)

Within these pillars of health, there are many ways to proceed towards your goals. Some people respond better than others to the various modalities. The goal is to build a foundation based on the principles above and then test and tweak to your preference. You don't have to be perfect; you just have to work consistently in the right direction. These things take time; they proceed slowly, inch by inch, day by day. You will not change years of bad habit in a day, week, or even year. It's like building a house; it takes one brick at a time. You must lay the foundation by strategically placing one brick and letting it dry rock-solid before placing another. Think of your habits like this: **stack good habit upon good habit.**

Your brain prefers the path of least resistance. It will resist your every effort. It will sabotage you, play tricks on you, give up on you, and be a lead weight weighing you down. We can combat this by starting with proper understanding that will lead to the right mindset. Once you get your brain in your corner, you will have a massive advantage. Work on making your brain your strongest asset instead of your biggest liability--like it is for most people.

You might notice that most of my emphasis isn't even relating to fitness or food recommendations. If you can't make yourself do the work, than what's the point of knowing any of the *how*? First and foremost, your **why** needs to be understood. Failing to understand your belief system, how you develop lasting habits, and the pitfalls lying in the weeds of your subconscious, will result in inevitable failure. Your mind dictates everything; it's the root of it all and you better get it in your corner.

The Current Industry

Most fitness advice is bland and most articles and books on these topics are boring. Usually, it's the same advice that has been regurgitated over and over. Fitness advice often sells hope and little in the way of result. It focuses too much on the *how* and completely misses the *why*. Yet still, people eat it up. People love to hope and desire but they don't like to do the work. They don't want to hear that they need to make sacrifices. They don't want to hear that they need to change their eating. They want the Magic Pill; the easy way out.

So what happens when reality sets in and hope fades? On to the next book, author, diet, or program. The grass-is-greener syndrome kicks in, and they hop from program to program and recommendation to recommendation in search of the "Promised Land." Their hope is revitalized with each new recommendation and they are again ready to give it a go. This lasts a few weeks, maybe a few months, until it all comes crashing down again; then on to the next program or pill or recommendation.

Why is this so prevalent? Is the average person really that blind when it comes to this stuff? YES! They are that blind, and dumb, and it's not entirely their fault. Let me explain. You see, weight-loss and body changes require a complete lifestyle shift to translate into real results. It's not as simple as a bit here or a bit there. If you want to crush some major goals, and make major changes, than you need to make a big shift in what you are doing. This lifestyle shift is only going to happen if the mind is 100% on board. It won't work if there is a shred of doubt in the subconscious. This shift also requires many factors that require cutting back on things we enjoy while also doing more of the things we don't. This is at odds with the lazy, stare at a screen, stay in-doors, work too much, sleep-deprived, and processed-food society that we live in today. Since we are so starved for time, and need a quick fix, we tend to look at our health as something we can solve if we just "get to the gym" or if we just "go on a diet." While both of these are integral to your fitness, they are only parts of the whole picture. And to further complicate this, there is little covered in popular literature that addresses the habits and beliefs that are necessary for long-term success.

As I keep harping on, your mindset is the key to success and gets near-zero exposure in the fitness industry. (There isn't much profit in showing people how to be successful on their own without the supplements, books, and thousands of redundant articles).

The Foundation of Health and Fitness

Break down the foundations of health further and we find that in each category there are hundreds of things you we can do right or royally fuck up. To exacerbate this, we have the fitness and food industries spitting out misinformation regarding what we should and shouldn't do. This marketing (propaganda) is how they get you to buy their shit (yes, the literal use of that word). And yes, they are winning. They have done a damn fine job of creating a consumer market that is misinformed, sick, and stuck in the cycle. This is why people are so dumb with this stuff. They are made so by the government, corporations, news, media, ads, quacks, etc.

I want you to see just how fucked up it is in the hopes that that you will have a fighting chance. I want you to see light where most are blind. Many of you need to "unlearn" everything you think you know. I'm going to plug two of my favorite authors here. These two are closer to the solution than anyone: Robb Wolf, author of "The Paleo Solution" and Mark Sisson from MarksDailyApple.com. I recommend you visit each of their websites and buy all of their books.

Take a breath. Open your mind.

It's time to let go of your previous mindset, and all the ideas and notions that came with it. You can trust me. I don't benefit if you take my advice or heed my warnings (other than knowing I helped saved another one). I hope to help you avoid becoming another statistic. I want you to start thinking differently and letting go of your limiting beliefs. I want you to see through the dogma that has been fed to you your entire life. I want you to seek the truth, ask questions, and come to your own conclusions. Either you will open your mind and start the process, or you will slip back under your warm, cozy blanket of denial. I truly want you to get there, to crush your goals and live a long, prosperous, and joyful life. But it is only going to happen if we have complete transparency with each other. You need to understand exactly what it takes and what you are getting yourself into. Understanding and accepting the challenges ahead is the key to mentally preparing yourself for success.

Ok, I think we are ready. Let's get to the single most important part of this complex system we call your health and fitness: **food**. Food is the most important thing, hands down. After food comes sleep and after that is fitness. Finally, we come to lifestyle and everything that it entails: stress reduction, rest, recovery, mindfulness, awareness, purpose, and balance.

Before diving into these specific subjects, you must understand that it will take a full commit to this lifestyle for the rest of your life. This is your health we are talking about here. It isn't a fad or a summer attempt at abs. It's the rest of your life and it's going to determine how long—and the quality–that life is going to be. This is some serious shit. Make sure you are on board with this fact.

To finish out with this long introduction, I'm leaving you with a few motivational paragraphs. The rest of this book is composed of single topic articles on specific ideas that I have been writing and meditating on for the last 8 years. These chapters were originally featured on AGymLife.com and have been edited or expanded where necessary. Check out AGymLife.com and subscribe to my list to stay up to date with my new essays. If you have any questions, comments, or feedback, shoot me an email: ismynamecolin@gmail.com

Remember: It's going to take commitment and a ton of hard work but you will absolutely get there if you stay the course.

The secret to living a long healthy life with a body you are proud of: Eat whole natural food, sleep 8 hours a night, move often, engage in high-intensity exercise a few times a week, lift heavy things, hang with friends and family, believe in something, have purpose in your work, and quiet your mind of worry, dread, fear, anxiety, and apprehension.

Translate this into action: Get moving, skip dessert, skip your next meal all together, clean your pantry out, go workout, do 100 push-ups, do 100 sit-ups after the push-ups, go for a walk, read a book, turn your phone off, get outdoors, play a sport, get some sun, slow cook a meal, cook a meal, go outside and sprint as far as you can, get on the ground and stretch, do yoga, hike, climb, row, run, swim, play, and most importantly, enjoy the process.

My Philosophy By Colin Stuckert

I believe that health and time are our most valuable resources.

Food, exercise, and mental awareness are the modalities I use to improve my health and longevity. I want to avoid hospitals, doctors, and dentists. I want to increase my chances of survival so I can better provide for my family.

As my health improves, I am granted more time and a better body to enjoy life with. With optimal health and abundant time I can do what I want, when I want, for as long as I want.

Each day I wake, I want to feel great and live that day to the fullest. I will balance my goals with living in the now and appreciating what I have instead of worrying about what I don't. I will remind myself that fulfillment is internal, a choice. If I choose contentment, everything else is a bonus. And most important of all, I can't seek true contentment if my health is fucked up.

This is my definition of freedom. And it is worth more to me than all the riches in the world.

"How To Live Life" By Colin Stuckert

Life each day to the fullest.

When you do something, do it deliberately and to the best of your ability.

When you love, love with everything.

When you laugh, laugh hearty.

When you eat, savor every bite.

When life doesn't go your way, accept the challenge and overcome.

When you suffer loss, mourn then heal.

When others harm you, forgive them.

When you make mistakes, learn from them and forgive yourself.

When you give, give without expectation.

Live as if each day was your last, because it is: there is no guarantee of tomorrow.

If you wake up tomorrow remember: you have been given a gift, the gift of life. Savor it each second of each day for as long as you are fortunate enough to receive it.

Results Getting

Results getting is easy and hard. It's easy because the formula is right in front of your face. You have limitless resources that show you how to squat, eat, cook, and so on. The Internet is overloaded with how-to information that makes the implementation part a breeze. That's the good news. The bad news is it's very hard to develop the habits necessary, control your urges, and fight your brain's inclination to take the path of least resistance. There are a plethora of pitfalls to fall into; all of which want to keep you fat, sick, and plugged into the matrix as a blind consumer. The only way to combat these dangers is to develop your mindset through awareness and knowledge.

Mindset is everything

Your mind controls everything in your life. It determines if you are happy, sad, worried, or afraid. It dictates everything you do and don't do. It is your reality for better or worse. Mindset is the most difficult aspect of reaching your goals because you—as a human being—are notoriously bad at understanding yourself and controlling the thoughts that go through your head. Most people go through life avoiding pain and pursuing pleasure; this is blindness. They never take the time to truly understand what they want or how they feel about life. This creates an internal unsettledness that festers and creates discontent. I want you to understand the importance of this topic. This work must be started now; it's going to be the hardest thing you've ever done. As you train your mind, your habits will get better. You will become more efficient at doing what needs to be done and results will creep up. As you continue on this path, you will see more results and your habits will become more automatic as a result. This is the ticket--*making these habits automatic*.

A Basic Template For Fitness:

1. Weightlifting: Lift weights at least 3 times a week. Focus on the big lifts: deadlift, squat, bench press, press, cleans, jerks, snatches. Focus on the compound accessory movements: pull-ups, dips, push-ups, pistols, one-arm PU/PU, plyometrics, kettlebell swings, etc.

2. Conditioning: Sprint, carry, lift, drag and throw heavy shit. Run long distance sometimes, row, swim, bike, play sports, don't use the elliptical, and forget the treadmill (get outside).

3. Follow a program template or listen to your body and train it hard every time you step foot in the gym. Those with specific goals should follow a legitimate program focused on that specialty. A general GPP program can do wonders for 99% of you. I recommend a general GPP program and Starting Strength or 5/3/1 for your strength program.

4. Make sure you rest: Most trainees should utilize two full rest days every week. Some will need more. For those that hate resting, you can spend time on active recovery: yoga, walking, hiking, and other low-impact physical activity. Remember, rest is where your body repairs and gets stronger and it should not be neglected.

5. Eat a clean diet with lots of high-quality protein and fat. Eat low-carb consisting of starchy veggies, some fruit, yams, and sweet potatoes. Athletes should use slightly higher carbs as determined by activity level.

6. Manage lifestyle factors: Sleep, stress, recovery, etc.

That's it. Don't complicate it. Don't let your lack of understanding hold you back. You don't need to understand WHY these things work; they do, so shut up and get doing. Don't get bogged down by *paralysis by analysis*. Needing to know everything is just going to slow your results getting. If you take the 6 steps listed above, and put in work for each one, you will see results. *I absolutely guarantee it.*

You know what you need to do and you have the resources you need to do it... now get to the hardest part of it all: **DOING**. Get doing. Get working. Let me know if you need any help or support along the way. I'm here to help.

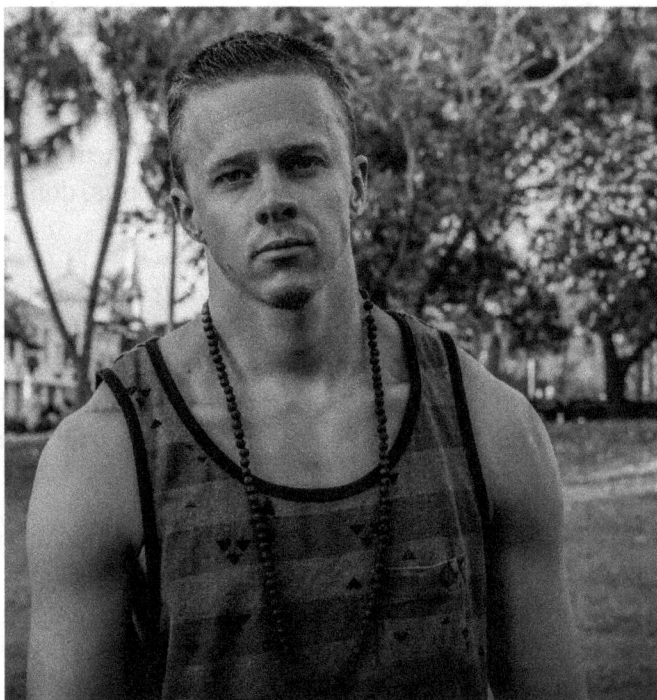

Yours in Fitness,

-Colin Stuckert

P.S. Hop on my mailing list and get the Sunday Gym Life emails as well as all my new work as it comes out. www.GymLifeClub.com

The Manifesto

The Gym Life is about better.

It is a lifestyle rooted in becoming better. It's not about being the best, just better than before, better than yesterday. It's a journey and a practice. No matter where you are, or where you want to be, you are always trying to become a better you.

This is the Gym Life Manifesto

The gym is a tool we use to improve physically as well as a place that signifies our seeking of better. It isn't the only thing, but it is integral in our lives. It's not just a means to an end either. It is a practice, like meditation. The work we do in the gym develops our body and mind. It is who we are. We will train until the day we die.

Our seeking of better is rooted in the inner belief that life is to be savored because it is precious and short. We won't squander this gift that has been granted to us by a higher power (god or nature, whichever you believe).

We have a yearning for more from life. We believe in experiences, relationships, and living an exceptional life. Our body and mind are one and we train them accordingly. The gym, what we eat, and how we live are a reflection of our goals to do more, be more, and see more. These routines enable us to live the best life possible. They grant us enjoyment in the present, time in the future, and a greater quality of life doing both.

We are passionate people. This passion seeps into our lives and is infectious to others. Others ask us how we do it and praise our dedication. We gladly lend a helping hand because we want to share our passion with others and we want the world to be a better, healthier place.

We are seekers of the truth. We enjoy new research that allows us to train, eat, and live better. We are not closed-minded; we can't be or we would regress. We are always learning and evolving and we love the process, it keeps life exciting.

Open-minded, yet analytical, we will give anything a change and then make an educated decision. We won't waste time trying to convince others. We offer what has worked for us and nothing more. We leave the debating to the Internet trolls. We are thinkers and doers, not talkers.

We know that our mind is our greatest asset. So we sharpen it to a fine edge. Research, questioning, and listening are the tools we use to increase our knowledge of the world, and more importantly, ourselves.

We try to understand our motivations. We live in a state of regular restraint and understand the importance that the subconscious plays in staying the course. We know that control of our mind is control of our bodies.

Ultimately, we seek happiness.

We believe that the key to achieving happiness is rooted in our mind. Training is a practice that helps us achieve great things and become self-aware. We are the seekers of truth in a way, the truth of our selves. We have found that our Truth is to live in our own reality and shape it so that the world is a guest and not vice versa.

We aim to become comfortable with being uncomfortable. We actively do things to push ourselves mentally and physically out of our comfort zones. That is how we grow and we know it is the only way.

We say fuck comfort. Forget what's easy. Life is short, get moving...

Join me...

-Colin Stuckert

What you should know about me

I started The Training Box 6 years ago. I've been training, coaching, eating, cooking, sleeping, and enjoying the ride since then. I've learned a ton and still do everyday.

My life philosophy

Death can come any moment and tomorrow isn't a guarantee. Think about that the next time you hesitate on something. Consider it as you watch another opportunity pass you by. Remember it the next time your stubbornness keeps you from sharing your feelings with someone you love. Remind yourself that the next time you hold back from saying sorry.

We are only specks of dust in the grand design of the universe and time. Why not make the most of it? Ultimately, no one is going to care either way. You might as well enjoy the ride. At the end of your life, no one will remember your failures, your mistakes, or your shortcomings. They will remember the art you made and the lives you touched. On the flip side, you will remember your failures, mistakes, and shortcomings if you give them the power. You will have regrets if you give them power. You will live a life for others if you give others power.

I implore you: live for yourself

Don't give anyone or anything power over you. At the end, you will realize how stupid you were to not act, or to care what others thought. Don't wait till you are old and gray to take chances. Don't wait until you are dying to be *ready*. Don't wait until the end to look back regretfully. As Epictetus said, "If you want to improve be content to be thought foolish and stupid."

Start living every day as if it were your last. Put more emphasis into your relationships and experiences. Help others as often as you can. Be weary of chasing money, fame, power, or tangibles. Fuck comfort. Comfort is a killer. Start making yourself uncomfortable. Get in there and give them hell. Make a difference.

My writing manifesto

I write so you can take action and better yourself. I spend a lot of time, and write a lot of words, in hopes that your mindset will be affected. And maybe, hopefully, you will understand on a level deep enough to elicit a physical response in you, one that moves you towards doing. I'm hoping to plant a seed in your subconscious that will start you making wiser decisions. Eventually, as this seed grows into a nagging weed, you will become more conscious and make better decisions as a result. The ultimate goal is for your every decision to be informed, and for you to attain absolute control of your life, your results, and your happiness. *That's what I hope for.* As you make more and more changes to your behavior, your results will start to creep in. **That's what I want for you—Results.** I want you to create inner changes that lead to a better, healthier life.

I'm hoping to reach as many people as possible. I won't reach everyone, but I will still try. I want to make a dent in the mind of the people I'm able to reach. Like Steve Jobs said, "I want to make a dent in the universe."

Ultimately, the only thing that matters is that you learn something to make yourself better. I want to hear: **"I'm doing."** That is my reward. To me, a writer is a vessel to transport ideas into the minds of others. I'm not a prophet or a preacher. My ideas are drawn from my life, my experiences, and what I have learned. I want you to read these words, absorb something actionable, and then act. Then, hopefully, these ideas will grow like a weed in your subconscious into a garden of conscious right actions.

Maybe this sounds audacious and a bit delusional; well, I think that's exactly what it's going to take. I might as well try to change the world and be happy changing a few lives along the way. The effort is the same and message will be the same.

I believe mindset is everything. To change the world, you must first believe that you can. The same goes with your life. To change your life, you must believe that you can beyond any doubt. You must destroy any negative self-talk or limiting beliefs that are holding you back. Many of you are sick, lost, and dying a slow death. Some of you are already working hard, some of you don't care, and some of you are "going to start next week." Either way, many of you need simple-to-implement advice that can get you headed in the right direction. I'm here to help you with that.

Healthy people don't buy drugs, see doctors, eat processed food, or consume 'miracle' supplements. I aim to help dispel the BS that surrounds these topics. When it comes to your health and fitness: *Knowledge really is power and ignorance really is killing you.*

And then we have the fitness industry….

There is so much crap in my profession. I'm sick of seeing the bias studies—if you can even call them that—that *conveniently* reach the goal they funded the study to reach; pure bias crap. Aren't we all sick of the blogs that write vanilla articles about the same shit that has been published a thousand times? What about those list posts that include the same "tips" that have been published by every wanna-be blogger in the world? I'm sick of those BS 'The Best Foods For' pieces. Those are the worst.

ATTENTION: There isn't any magic fruit or vegetable that's going to save your life. You want to know what the best food is? Organ meats. When did you see an article encouraging you to eat more liver? Really, give me a break. BTW, you're welcome—I just saved you from having to read the next 100 articles about why green veggies are good for you because they contain some vitamins and minerals and vitamins and minerals are good for you because they are good. Think about it: The amount of nutrition in a grass-fed steak or salmon fillet completely demolishes an equal amount of any green veggie. You would have to eat POUNDS of spinach to equal a few bites of healthy animal meat. **POUNDS.** You know what a pound of greens looks like? Yea, it's the veggie section, the entire section. Don't waste your time on mainstream nutrition, health, and fitness writing. Most of it is pure crap.

Disclaimer=I still recommend fruits and vegetables because they are a great way to replace junk food and they do provide nutritional value when consumed in colorful in-season variety. I'm not discrediting veggies or fruit; I'm just calling-out the emphasis on them and how people think they are the best things you can eat. The best thing you can eat is a healthy animal. Period.

I'm also sick of the countless articles on lifting weights that promises the next breakthrough that is going to get you "jacked."

Try this: get in the gym and do sets of reps until you can't do anymore.

Wow, what a novel concept? I just saved you from reading the next 150,000 articles on Tnation. Do you really think Arnold and the huge dudes in the 70s followed some fad program? They just squatted, deadlifted, and put heavy shit overhead as often as they physically could. **It's easy: move heavy weight up repeatedly, train hard, and rest between efforts.** Listen to your body. That's it. It isn't rocket science.

What about conditioning?

Conditioning is another easy formula for the majority of you: Mix it up among different modalities: Strongman, swimming, biking, running, sprinting, intervals, Tabata. Go short and intense most of the time, medium distance sometimes, and long distance every so often. Walk a lot. Listen to your body.

That's it. I just gave you the formula that could cripple a billion dollar information industry. No more books, magazines, or articles, just people following a 1-page template that works. This is exactly what the 99% should be doing. And make no mistake, I say this all as an optimist. I'm fighting what I call *the good fight* by arming you with knowledge so you can have a fighting chance against all the BS out there. When the playing field is level, you can choose to be a lazy fat-ass if you want and that is your right. I will rest easy knowing I did all I could. Unfortunately, the field isn't level and it screws a lot of good people up. *This is my mission: To make fitness, food, and living a healthy life easy to understand.*

Here is the basic formula for reaching your goals:

• Eat real food • Eat less frequently (skip meals, eat fewer meals throughout the day) • Train hard a few times a week (lift weights + condition) • Walk and move a lot • Sleep 8 hours • Reduce stress anyway possible • Believe in something and have a purpose • Have relationships.

Within each of these categories there are many paths to take and many modalities to train. You should get as good as you can in each one. Start today. Use YouTube, AGymLife.com, coaches at your box, or your friendly local athlete to help you in each category. Ask for advice, practice, and get better on a daily basis. It won't happen overnight; it's a journey. The only thing that matters is that you start and never stop.

Fitness is an education, like a martial art, and you must progress through the ranks in knowledge and technique. We all start as white belts and eventually we can become black belts with enough effort. When you are armed with the right information, and you implement hard, you can get there. But the more BS you are fed, the longer it is going to take. The more diets you try or programs you hop, the longer it is going to take. For me, it has been a long, hard road. My white belt to black belt journey has been raging on for the last 11 years since I first stepped foot into a Gold's gym. If I knew what I now know, I'd probably be doing something completely different with my life. My struggle on this journey has led me to develop a passion (more like an obsession) for food and fitness. Life is funny like that. And I want to pass on the knowledge I've gained over the years to you.

Your time is now. Get healthy. Get moving. No excuses.

50 Ways To Lose Weight

The subject of this chapter is losing weight but it also doubles as a guide on how to live a healthy lifestyle. Overall, you u will lead a better life if you make your lifestyle look something like 1 through 20. Following 21-50 will help you lose weight *and* improve whatever you are training towards. Pick and choose tips that resonate with you while focusing on dialing in 1 through 20 as the baseline.

1. Eat a grain-free Paleo/Primal diet. Health and longevity are centered on eating foods that resemble a Paleo diet (unprocessed, from nature). If you can't go 100% grain-free Paleo you should, at the very least, be eating unprocessed whole foods straight from nature.

Food is fuel. Only ingest the highest quality fuel you can find. Weight loss becomes effortless when you are eating real food.

2. Get lots of sleep. I have clients that look at me sideways when I tell them they need to sleep 8+ hours a night. If you are one of these sleep-deprived zombies, I challenge you to try it for a week. You will be amazed by how you feel and where your body composition goes with this little experiment. You may realize that you have been in a chronic state of sleep deprivation your entire life.

3. Practice intermittent fasting (IF)/Eat less often. I follow the leangains.com approach: A daily 8-hour feeding window followed by a 16-hour fast. Whether you follow a strict fasting protocol or not, you can definitely benefit from skipping meals on a regular basis. Contrary to popular belief, skipping meals can help you build muscle (it also provides a ton of other health-related benefit).

4. Eat slow and chew your food thoroughly. This has done **wonders** for me. I used to inhale food like a whale gobbling up plankton. I would just swim right through the food until it was gone in a matter of seconds. Eating slow enables some important triggers for weight loss:

1. You reduce the insulin spike by slowing the release of glucose into your blood stream. This prevents insulin, a storage hormone, from storing calories in your fat cells—more insulin = more fat storage.

2. You eat less. Eating slow makes you feel full faster and avoid taking in extra calories. We all hate that full, bloated feeling. That is the result of eating too fast and not allowing the *full* trigger enough time to tell your brain to PUT DOWN THE DAMN FORK.

5. Cook your food at home. Restaurant food is bad. Restaurants use cheap salt, sugar, sauces, thickeners, stabilizers and all kinds of other unnatural crap to reduce costs, stay profitable, and keep the food addictive. The average restaurant margin is well under 5%; it's a tough business. You better believe they do everything they can to cut corners and save on food costs, and when this happens, the customer is the one that gets stuck with the health bill.

6. Don't drink calories. When my clients cut out soda/juices/beer they usually see 5+ pound weight-loss results within the first week. Drinking calories elicits a similar negative response on insulin levels that eating your food too fast does. The calories enter your blood stream too quickly and cause an overload of insulin. We are made to chew our food. Avoid drinking calories in any form.

7. Go completely gluten-free. This can be life changing. Clean out your pantry and be super-picky when eating out (say no to the free bread). This could be the missing link to that lean body you've been trying to achieve.

8. Don't snack. Snacking is the bane of weight loss. One of the reasons intermittent fasting is so beneficial is because it regulates your hormone levels by balancing your body between the fasted and fed states. Basically, your body is made to burn fat when in the 'fasted' state and made to store calories when in the 'fed' state. Every time you put calories in your mouth you are entering the 'fed' state and thus shutting off your bodies ability to burn fat by introducing glucose and insulin into your blood stream.

Next time you grab that bag of almonds thinking it's a healthy snack, you should think again: you are actually doing your body a disservice. Eat only during your meal times.

9. Take high quality fish oil (or cod liver oil) with every meal. Fish oil contains omega-3's that help to balance out the omega-6's that are prevalent throughout our modern diets (especially processed foods). Correcting this balance provides a major benefit to the body, especially weight loss. My favorite brands are Carlson and Natural Stacks.

10. Take vitamin D or get sunlight everyday. This could be the missing link in your weight loss program. Vitamin D is a necessary hormone in the human body. It is too damn important in too many processes in your body to neglect. Take a vitamin D soft-gel or get 20 minutes of sunlight every day.

11. Reduce stress at all costs. Do everything you can to reduce and avoid stress. Every time you get angry, stressed, or freak-out about something it is like taking a bite out of a candy bar. Stress releases cortisol and insulin into your blood stream just like taking a bite of your favorite candy bar. As we discussed earlier, the extra release of insulin halts fat-loss and promotes fat-gain (cortisol also messes shit up). That's a bad combination don't you think? Take a chill pill and BREATHE.

12. Practice mindfulness. Mindfulness is the act of focusing on a single object or task and turning off the rest of the noise (thoughts, worry, stress) going through your head. This helps with number 11 in lowering and preventing chronically raised cortisol and insulin levels. Our hormones get all out of whack as a result of our mind tormenting us with worry, stress, anger, resentment, jealously, and all kinds of other shit we shouldn't be worrying about.

Some techniques for being mindful: Counting your breath (breath meditation), sitting in a quiet place with the goal of emptying the mind (meditation), going outdoors and focusing on the sights and sounds while tuning out the rest of your life. Listen, I'm not a pro here, just a student, so I suggest you do more research on your own. A little practice goes a long way. Recommended books: The Power of Now, Zen Mind, Beginner's Mind.

13. Eliminate sugar. It's the absolute worst thing you can eat. Remember that fat doesn't make you fat. Sugar, seed oils, and processed grains are what make you fat

14. Eat lots of high-quality fat. Fatty fish, grass-fed beef, lamb, bison, coconut oil, olive oil (I prefer it unheated), Kerrygold butter, avocado oil, macadamia oil, ghee, lard (make your own), tallow (make your own).

15. Eat lots of high-quality animal products. Keywords include: grass-fed, free range, pastured, organic, all-natural, hormone-free, humanely raised, family farms, local.

16. Perform resistance training ~3 times a week. You probably already know why this is beneficial. Just do it.

17. Perform high-intensity conditioning ~3 times a week. Think intervals: short, fast, and hard. Avoid long distance and moderate paced training as the bulk of your training (it's only useful sometimes).

18. Walk Everywhere. Take the stairs, park at the end of the parking lot, and always take the long way. We are made to move at a slow pace frequently. Get up and get moving.

19. Play sports. Sports are great for overall health, mental relief, muscle building, mobility, social development, etc. We have been playing games since the dawn of man.

20. Get outdoors as much as possible. It's good for so many reasons.

The first 20 are the fundamentals to living a healthy life. As you adopt more and more of this list, you will notice that you become a fat-burning machine, and you'll soon realize how easy it is to tweak your weight based on what you do or don't do. I recommend you incorporate these habits a little at a time until they become routine. Don't try to adopt them all at once or you will probably get frustrated and fail.

21. Drink a full glass of water before each meal. You will feel full faster and eat less.

22. Eat your protein before your carbs and fat. Protein is very satiating and will fill you up fast.

23. Eat a bit of healthy fat 15 minutes before each meal. Fat curbs appetite and triggers the release of hormones that let you know you are full. You can kick start these hormones by nibbling on some nuts or dark chocolate before your meals.

24. Eat hot and hearty soups and stews. Soups and stews are filling. Eat them HOT and slow (prevents overeating).

25. Sprint. Fast, intense, full-body exercise like sprinting has insane thermogenic and EPOC effects on the body. Basically, it turns your body into a calorie-burning furnace. Sprinting also builds massive muscle (compare a pic of a sprinter to a marathon runner, it's scary).

26. Make things difficult for yourself, on purpose. Why would you ever do this? So you can move more, DUH! The more movement you perform, the more calories you burn. Instead of always taking the easiest route, try this: grit your pussy willow lip and get moving.

27. Buy some Chuck Taylors or Oly shoes. You will lift more and the more weight you move, the more calories you burn and muscle you build.

28. Drink green tea. It's full of antioxidants and a bit of caffeine, both good for fat burning.

29. Chew a few extra chews each mouthful. Chewing has been linked to improvement in digestion and breakdown of food through the release of the saliva enzymes amylase (starch breakdown) and lipase (fat breakdown).

30. Drink black coffee (in moderation). Coffee offers many benefits to the body, one of which is fat burning, but there are some caveats. You should drink black and organic if possible (or try Bulletproof coffee, it's amazing). Only buy the best beans, they are one of the most heavily sprayed crops in the world.

31. Take a digestive enzyme, probiotic, and/or eat fermented food regularly. These products improve gut health and digestion. The better you digest your food, the better it is utilized in the body and the less likely it will be converted into adipose tissue. Adipose tissue is FAT ladies and gentlemen, the jiggley, cellulitely, unpleasant kind of fat.

32. Perform heavy, complex, functional movements. Anything that trains the body as a whole is going to eat up calories for fuel. If you are stuck in *isolation-land*, I implore you to start picking up, carrying, and moving heavy shit on a regular basis. Go big and compound or go home.

33. Avoid liquid food. And yes, that includes protein shakes. You should avoid liquid calories in any form if you are trying to lose weight. We know that drinking calories produces a large insulin spike and we also know that insulin is a storage hormone that signals our body to store calories. Well, do you know where those calories get stored? Yup, as fat.

Disclaimer: If you drink a shake in lieu of eating a meal, then I say it's not that bad as long as you keep it simple and low-carb. Avoid those 500-calorie oat, peanut butter, and fruit smoothie concoctions (those are for weight gain). If it keeps you from eating shit and you want to drink a shake, then stick with water and whey and drink it slow.

34. Skip the condiments. How did I lose 10 pounds and finally carve out my abs after 2 years of frustration? Dropping ketchup (I also nixed milk). I used to drown my chicken breasts in ketchup; they were swimming. Eliminating this single product allowed me to bust through a stubborn plateau. Store-bought condiments are filled with sugar and other processed crap. There is no reason to include them in your diet, especially considering how easy it is to substitute with homemade or organic options. These seemingly small changes are what separate those that have abs and those who don't.

35. Drink lots of water. You don't need to drink as much water as the pundits would have you believe, but for reducing cravings and making us feel full more often, water can be useful. Listen to your thirst; it's there for a reason.

36. Think hard - Use your brain. Your brain's primary fuel source is glucose, so obviously it is beneficial to use up as much of it as possible so there isn't any leftover to be stored as fat.

37. Perform Tabata intervals. A Tabata interval is 20 seconds of work followed by 10 seconds of rest. Pick a movement—Air squat for example—and start a timer. Perform as many air squats in 20 seconds as possible, and then rest. Go again after 10 seconds of rest. Repeat until 4 minutes is up and 8 rounds have been completed. The Tabata Interval is a brutal, effective, and simple exercise protocol that you can do with any exercise or movement.

38. Replace soda, juice, and sweet tea with a soda water and lime (sparkling and seltzer also work). This is how my sister and I weaned off soda (a long time ago mind you). It allowed us to satisfy that craving for carbonation without the calories or sugar. You can even fake it at the club with a soda water and lime—you will still look *super-cool* and no one will know you are sipping carbonated water.

39. Do NOTHING. Relieve stress by turning off your brain and laying around like a fat-lazy Jabba the Hutt from time to time. This is something some of us do well (or too much) and others do terribly (never relax). Examples of doing nothing include: watching mindless

TV, movies, people watching, lying on the beach, napping, and so on.

40. Take naps. Sleep is one of the top 5 techniques to living a healthy life. Naps consist of sleep. Thus, naps do a body good (milk does not).

41. Get social. Humans are social animals that have survived for thousands of by staying together. The benefits of enjoying time with friends and family are enormous. Anything that improves happiness and makes us feel good will help us lose weight by reducing stress.

42. Fast before you train. The longer you go without food in your body the more you will burn stored fat. Training increases your body's need for fuel. Your body will utilize fat stores for fuel if there is a lack of glucose in your blood stream. Fasting helps keep glucose out of your bloodstream so your body can burn off fat instead.

43. Watch your carb intake. This includes sugar, rice, potatoes, fruit, and grains (hopefully no grains). Even *good* carbs can become *bad* if you eat too much of them.

44. Take ZMA before bed (Zinc, Magnesium & Vitamin B-6). ZMA is hands down my favorite supplement. Magnesium aids in weight loss and is beneficial to a host of other body functions; one of which is improved sleep. You will sleep deeper, fuller, and longer. This should be a standard supplement in your program.

45. Do HIIT. Seriously, everyone can and should do some form of HIIT programming. You can do more WODs, Less WODs, strength-bias, endurance-bias, gymnastics-bias, powerlifting-bias, etc. If you've never tried HIIT training, I highly suggest finding a local affiliate and trying a free class.

46. Utilize active-rest days. Those days where you can barely walk and your back feels like a giant bruise (I heart that feeling) are days that you should avoid training. This is the perfect time for an active rest day.

An active rest day: work mobility, do some light rowing and jogging, work on Oly technique with an empty barbell, foam roll, stretch, and so on.

Go at a slow and easy, yet deliberate, pace. This will improve recovery, reduce stress on your body, help recover your CNS, and get your body moving. This also improves fat burning and muscle building.

47. Go for gluten-free hard cider over gluten-filled beer and opt for liquor and soda water over sugar-filled mix drinks. Beer and mixed drinks are the Antichrist to your abs. A long Island ice tea has 780 calories and about 40 grams of sugar. I used to drink those [Smacks forehead].

48. Avoid artificial sweeteners. This includes splenda, aspartame, and other 'naturally flavored' sweeteners. Sweeteners spike your insulin levels because your brain can't tell the difference between them and sugar. Thus the body response ends up being the same. They also probably cause cancer. It just makes sense to avoid them. *Stevia is ok but I would still go light.

49. Don't overtrain. Avoid overtraining at all costs. It saps weight-loss efforts and promotes fat-gain via the huge amounts of cortisol release that causes havoc in your body.

50. Plan ahead/pack a lunch. The best way to avoid falling off the wagon and eating junk is to be prepared. Always have something healthy with you. One-pot meals are great for being prepared throughout the week.

How to Implement (the most important part)

Step 1: Be patient. Your new habits will take time to implement and time for the results to show. The people who get shit done in life are the one's who stay the course. Stay the damn course.

Step 2: Test, Tweak, Test, Tweak

You must test and tweak on a regular basis to find the right combination that works for you. All of these techniques will work for everyone to varying degrees if implemented in their purest forms, however, the dose and result can be vary wildly from person to person. No matter what, we will always be learning, growing, and improving if we put in the effort. Now get your ass in gear and get working!

Starting a Program

A Training program is a major life commitment. You had better be mentally "all-in" before you hop into a new fitness program or you aren't going to last. It's just the way it is. Remember, in this industry, the odds of people that get results is very, very low.

Whether you are just about to start a training program or already train consistently, the following points are important for long-term success with a program. So pay attention.

As Always: Mindset is Everything

Most programs have a high attrition rate because trainees have a hard time developing the habits necessary to stick with it. It isn't easy to train the body, eat clean, and live the holistic lifestyle necessary while simultaneously balancing work, stress, and our fast-paced society. It's a lot. It takes time to develop the habits that are necessary for long-term success. Research shows that it takes 21 days of effort to make a habit stick... at the minimum! It can take as much as 6 months for some people. Don't assume it's going to be easy.

Unfortunately, most people don't prepare themselves for the work ahead. They will give up after a few days and wonder why they never reach their goals. Each habit you develop into your routine is a mini-crusade in and of itself; and you should treat each one as the success that it is. If you can focus on accomplishing these small successes consistently, you will be much more motivated along the way and it will make the process that much easier. Then it will be just a matter of time.

Most new trainees jump into a program without any idea of what it takes to succeed. They have no plan, no guide, and no clue. Let's cover some basics of being successful with a training program.

1. You Need To Eat Clean. If you want that ripped or tone look, you **must** eat clean. There is no exception here. Nutrition will take your performance to incredible heights on top of making you look good. No one wants to be that girl or guy that looks-average-but-trains-4-days-a-week (and you see it all too often). It pains me to see trainees who don't have the body composition they should have. Fitness is about being functional and a byproduct of being functional is having a six-pack. If you consider yourself "fit," than you should have a six-pack. Period. If you don't have a six-pack, you have no one to blame but yourself. You need to fix your diet, sleep more, and stress less (and probably drink less).

So how do we eat clean? Easy: go gluten-free Paleo/Primal. It will change your life and give you a six-pack. Nutrition is one of the most important aspects of your body composition and health. Make it a priority now and it will pay dividends for the rest of your life.

2. Train Smart and Work Mobility. Training is very hard on the body. In fact, for some people, the volume and lack of recovery focus is a huge gap in their training program. Too many trainees try to follow programs used by elite athletes. This is a huge mistake, especially if your recovery sucks. To think that every person can train the same way, using the same workouts, on the same schedule, or with the same weights, is *absolutely ludicrous*. Yet, I see this all the time in my business and with the box gyms that are popping up left and right and attracting new trainees every day. They, and many others, miss the point of individual-based coaching, rest periods, and intelligent programming. You must scale, listen to your body, and use the least effective dose to reach your goals; not the dose that others use. Fitness is an individual pursuit through and through.

Athletes that eat crap, forgo supplements, and skip work on their mobility and stress-maintenance, cannot sustain long-term high-intensity training. And still, I see this all the time in my business. Breakdown of your joints is inevitable, overuse injuries are inevitable, and stress will always win as you continually break down your body and not give it due rest. You must respect what goes on outside of the gym as paramount in your results. Be smart with your training volume by making sure you schedule rest and recovery protocols as an integral part of your program.

Mobility work should be integral in your routine. Get a Foam Roller and roll out before and after your workouts. Lacrosse Balls are great for targeting trigger points in your back, glutes, and hips. Work on static stretches post-workout and dynamic mobility before.

3. Work on Active Recovery. Active recovery can be defined as engaging in recovery enhancing activities such as ice baths, hot water immersion, Epsom salt baths, self-massage, massage, walking, mobility, supplementation, and proper nutrition. Ice baths in short intervals (under 10 minutes) have shown to improve recovery. The same goes for hot water treatments. When recovering from physical activity, walking, jogging, and light movement have shown to speed up recovery as well.

4. You Need to Stay Consistent. I've owned The Training Box for 6 years now and it's depressing to see the amount of clients that sign-up, come for a month, and pay for 5 months of their 6 month contract without ever showing up again. This is a routine I see far more than I would like to admit and it sucks royally. It's quite telling of the psychology behind new trainees and how motivation can wax and wane. For new trainees, motivation is always high to start. Then, when motivation wanes and reality sets in, they realize how difficult it is to come in and train 3-4 days a week and to break their lazy, unhealthy habits. Then what happens is it all comes crashing down: They come less and less until eventually not at all. It's a bloody shame.

One reason their commitment breaks down is trainees fall into an "All or Nothing" mentally. They convince themselves that they must come to the gym 3 or 4 days a week or not at all. Isn't one day a week better than ZERO days a week? They fail to realize that a little bit goes a long way. The secret sauce is consistency, whether that is once a week or 5 times a week. The beauty of training is its effectiveness. One day a week is 100% better than zero days a week (duh). The same goes for two days a week over one day. Surprisingly, for 99% of the population who train to improve general body composition, two days a week is ample training to make steady gains.

Let's reiterate that: Twice a week of high intensity training is enough to make steady gains. That is only two hours of the 168 hours in your week, ladies and gents. Are your health and a sexy bod not worth that pathetically minimal investment? Excuses about why you don't have time are complete and utter nonsense. Anything in life worth having takes effort. The process is to be respected and the reward savored. If a ripped physique was easy to achieve no one would appreciate it and everyone would have it. It would be common and thus nothing special. Different, unique, and rare are sought after for a reason: because common is boring and readily available. You must decide if you want to be like everyone else (fat, lazy, and sick) or unique (ripped, sexy, strong, and original).

5. You Must Sleep 8+ Hours A Night. Sleep is one of the most important things we do as human beings. Do it right, do it consistently, and don't skimp. There is no shortcut here.

6. You Must Take a Rest Week Every Couple of Months. I see this ALL THE TIME in my box: athletes hit plateaus, they get sick, and their numbers degrade. I recommend a rest week when this happens. Your body will tell you when you need rest, so listen to it. It will slow down, you will feel weak, your PR's will lack. It's time for a rest week when this happens.

Conclusion

A training program is hard to stick to mentally and physically. It requires you to juggle many things simultaneously. It requires you to develop healthy habits while balancing your job, family, kids, school, and so on. It's not easy, by any means. But you can do it. You can balance it all and be successful.

Success comes from developing these habits for the long term. Most give up when they fail to develop the habits because it is just too hard to stay consistent through sheer willpower—you are human aren't you? It's against human nature to consciously force ourselves into painful situations, but you have to do it. You have to develop a passion for your training and nutrition. Make yourself uncomfortable and recognize that feeling as accomplishment. Then relish in it.

Your results come from top-notch nutrition, recovery, and rest habits.

Because of the difficulty in changing habits and lifestyle, the majority of people who start a program fail to stick with it. The way to succeed is to develop your habits. Start with one habit at a time. Each new habit change will have a complementary effect on your other habits. The more *good* habits you solidify into your routine, the easier it will be to change your *bad* habits. Eventually, you will end up with the majority of your habits falling into the "good" category.

And most important of all: Drop the all or nothing mentality. If you miss a few days, weeks, or months, that's ok, just focus on the NOW and <u>get your ass back in the gym</u>. Each new day is a chance to make a conscious decision for the better. This should always be independent of your past failures or future success. The only thing that matters is now. Get working now!

Why You Don't Get Results

The Magic Pill syndrome

A common mindset trap I see people fall into is what I call the "magic pill" syndrome. The magic pill syndrome varies from individual to individual but can be summarized as: wanting a shortcut to results.

In fitness this looks something like:

- Trying to buy results in the form of supplements, pills, etc.

- Trying to out-exercise a shitty diet (impossible)

- Trying to get six-pack abs but still get plastered each weekend (not gonna happen)

- Wishing for results long-term health yet unwilling to change lifestyle

For any result there must be the adequate input. This usually requires more than what most are willing to give or more than they realize is necessary. The difference between those that reach their goals and those that do not is a willingness to invest enough input—time, effort, consistency—to reach their goals. **Typically, an input requires time and effort. This equation looks something like this: Time (x) Habit = Result.**

If you invest enough time of a specific habit, you will see a result. Examples include sleeping, eating, abstaining from alcohol or drugs, etc. The result equation requires ONE dose of time and ONE dose of habit repeated over and over until you reach the end result. This is what we are shooting for: **the adequate dose for a long enough**

period of time. Most fall short before reaching their goals by missing a part of this equation.

In between these two spectrum ends you have something like: 1 * .5 = .5 ← Where .5 is represented as half time or half-effort. In this example, you reach only half way to your goal because you don't invest enough time or effort past a certain point. This is where the majority of results-seeking people are: **somewhere on the path to their results but not sure where**. The problem here is we are terrible judges of our results. We get frustrated; lose motivation, start eating crap, and end up making it way harder for ourselves. It's a constant yo-yo of motivation and strictness.

When we are moving towards a goal, we often get discouraged from feeling we have made little headway when in fact we may be doing everything right. To further compound this issue, we have hidden result indicators that take time to show positive results—eating clean as an example. You don't see the immediate benefits of eating better—although you will probably feel them. We might feel better but we don't see the internal changes and the external changes take time to show, sometimes a lot of it. This leads to frustration. We are impatient creatures who want what we want and now. This is at odds with results getting: it takes time.

To further compound this issue, most of us use the mirror to gauge our results. This is the most inaccurate measure of all, at least in the short term. Sometimes the mirror takes MONTHS to show the hard work paying off. The same goes for the scale. The internals of our body take time and are hidden from our view. It's simply too hard for most trainees to stay consistent until the results start showing. As a result, most give up before their results start to show.

Some ways to measure your results:

•A blood lipid test

•How you feel throughout the day

•Improved performance in the gym

- Better sex

- Better sleep – longer, fuller, deeper

- More happiness (tough to measure but possible)

- Less stress (same as happiness)

Some of the habits we need to stay consistent with are:

- Lifting heavy weights

- Frequent metabolic training

- Walking

- Eating slow

- Eating clean

- Staying gluten-free

- Drinking way less or not at all

- Sleeping 8 hours a night

- Meditation

How do we combat giving up?

First, you must accept what it is going to take: it's going to be a long, hard journey. In my experience, even a 60% adherence will provide results if you keep going. I recommend aiming higher than 60%, but as a starting point, anything above 50% is a great start and is usually enough to start showing positive changes. I recommend aiming for 80% adherence in all the variables: sleep, stress, training, diet, and lifestyle. It's unlikely you will ever reach 100% and that's ok. 80% will allow you to reach life-changing results and live a long and prosperous life. If you want to go above that than more power to you, but remember, the goal isn't perfection, it's progress.

Developing habits is tough work. The best way to develop a habit is to focus on only one habit at a time. Single-mindedly focus on it until it sticks. There are apps that help with this (like the app lift). Each habit you successfully implement will bring you that much closer to your goals. Keep in mind, though, that you want to build these habits into forever habits. You want to develop a routine that will last for the rest of your life. You are building a lifestyle that consists of a bunch of positive habits.

Think of your habits as the maintenance to the machine that is your body. If you neglect one or more, your results will systematically breakdown. When you reach your goals you will still need to maintain them. It is in your best interest to develop these habits now and get them to stick. Once you reach maintenance mode, this becomes a much simpler equation. But getting to this high level is still a huge journey.

Start working on your habits now... they will be with you forever

This might sound like a lot of work, but the reality is if we don't live a lifestyle that promotes the greatest expression of our genes (thanks to **Mark Sission** for this phrase) than we are broken. It is what it is folks. You want to strive for being as un-broken as possible. It comes back to the original point: nothing comes without the proper input.

There is no easy way. No free lunch. No magic pill. No secret program. **It all comes down to hard work and positive habit invested over a long enough period of time**.

So get working. Start building positive habits and get them working for you on a daily basis. Once you reach a high level of adherence, it gets much easier to maintain.

Remember: Time + Habit = you can accomplish anything!

What is the Paleo Diet?

The Paleo diet is a way of eating that replicates the diet of our ancestors who lived in the wild as hunter-gatherers before the creation of modern agriculture some 10,000 years ago. The Paleo diet consists of eating foods that are unprocessed and from nature—any "real" food, basically.

Grains, oats, rye, barley, beans, lentils, legumes, and synthetics are prohibited. These foods cause health issues and require processing to be consumable for humans because they are not edible in their raw, natural form. Any food that causes a negative response in the human body—the gut for example—is not one we should eat. Many of the foods that are not recommended on a Paleo diet cause gut issues like leaky gut, indigestion, and inflammation. When you avoid these foods, you avoid the stress to your body that eating these foods elicit. Additionally, when you replace them with foods that heal, you are adding a double benefit to your health and body. This double whammy of awesomeness is why so many people get extraordinary results after "going Paleo."

Preferred foods on a Paleo diet include healthy animals, vegetables, fruits, yams, nuts/seeds, and other editable raw foods from nature. These foods make up what really is <u>the human diet</u>. Eating real food from nature develops and repairs the human body while processed food negates health and causes internal damage. If a food requires processing, it is not human food—simple as that.

In a nutshell: Meat, Leaves, and Berries

The bulk of calories on a Paleo diet come from eating animals. Healthy animals provide the most nutrition per oz. than any other food on the planet. A colorful selection of in-season fruits and vegetables come next on the list. After that, we fill in the blanks with preferred starches such as yams, sweet potatoes, and squashes (white potatoes and white rice are considered Paleo but should be consumed in moderation because of their glycemic and carbohydrate loads). **The basic thesis is if it grew in nature, and has not been processed or altered, you can eat it.**

Foods excluded from the Paleo diet include grains, legumes, dairy, refined salt and sugar, processed oils, and other processed and artificial ingredients. If you read the label of any typical junk food item you will find many of these junk ingredients:

•**Brownie** = Grains, Dairy, Refined salt/sugar, processed oil

•**Candy** = Refined salt/sugar, artificial colorings and chemicals

•**Bread** = Grains, Refined salt/sugar, processed oil, artificial colorings and chemicals

•**Pasta** = Grains, Refined salt/sugar, processed oil, artificial colorings and chemicals

•**Most Restaurant Food** = Grains, legumes, Refined salt/sugar, processed oil, artificial colorings and chemicals

So Do I Starve Myself?

People are initially taken aback by the amount of options that aren't OK to eat. This shouldn't be a surprise considering most Americans follow a food pyramid that is completely backwards. Then, when I show them examples of the food I eat, they quickly realize that the options are plenty. The key to enjoying all that Paleo has to offer—and to staying consistent—is to avoid restaurants like the plague and focus on making home-cooked food using the best ingredients possible.

Why should I eat this way? Because your diet has made you sick and you are getting sicker; because our country is chronically sick, depressed, stressed, overworked, and missing out on a healthy life. And most importunately, because these problems are rooted in your poor food choices.

There is BIG BUSINESS in making and keeping us fat. Consider what happens when you get fat: You eat more food, drink more soda, need more drugs, watch more TV, crave more sugar, buy more fat-loss pills, and so on. What better business model than to sell food to people, get them hooked on it, and sell them more and more and more of what they don't need (looks a lot like the drug dealer business model, doesn't it?).

McDonald's is the largest fast-food chain in the world and they got that way using this exact formula. They use cheap-processed food to get millions addicted. Corporations such as Kraft, Monsanto, Tyson, and Perdue spend billions of dollars lobbying in Washington to ensure lax food regulations and encourage public misinformation through funding bias studies.

Cheap food comes with a price

Pay a few extra dollars in the grocery store or you will pay much more on the operating table. Complaining that it's too expense to eat healthy is pure ignorance. Food accounts for as high as 80% of a human beings health and longevity. How, please tell me, is it not the easiest, most clear-cut and obvious thing in the world to spend money on the best food possible and promote full-body health? It's a sick, stupid, and disgusting flip-flop of priorities we have grown accustomed to in this country. While other cultures sometimes spend half their paycheck on food or clean drinking water, we are so pathetically coddled that we complain about spending a few extra bucks on some grass-fed beef or organic veggies. Really?

The fact is it's not that much more expensive to buy better food, we are talking a few bucks here and there. If you are pressed for budget you can get creative and stretch your dollar. There are a million ways to buy quality food in large quantities (Costco, online, buy a whole cow). You can also utilize batch cooking to save time and get the most bang for your buck.

Recap

The Paleo diet is based on eating real food. Eating real food improves your health, betters the environment, improves the treatment of animals, and adds years to your life. Yes, you should feel guilty eating that processed crap, it promotes death and decay and you are supporting the company that profits from it. The next processed-bite you take should be coupled with a feeling of guilt, a feeling of weakness; a feeling that you are shaving years from your life and making the world a more terrible, pathetic, disgusting, and sick place. Is the temporary pleasure worth any or all of that? No, it isn't. So start the change. Start taking your food choices seriously.

We are made to eat and thrive on **REAL FOODS** found in **NATURE**. When you process food through heat, chemical or other means, you are removing the nature. Some foods, such as grains, are not meant to be consumed in their raw state at all and must undergo major heat processing to be edible for humans. This is a sign we are not meant to eat them!

No Processed anything: Grains, Legumes, Flour, Rye, Barley, Candy, Cake, Battered, Fried, etc.

All-Natural with Nothing-Added: Meat, Seafood, Veggies, Fruit, Potatoes, Yams, Nuts/seeds, Coconut, Pastured Butter

Benefits Of Paleo: You will lose weight. I have seen hundreds of clients in my gym adopt the Paleo way of eating and universally the following always happens:

They:

- Lose weight

- Lean up

- Get ripped

- Get stronger

- Feel better

- Sleep better

- Increase energy

- Have better sex

- Cure disease (no, I'm not exaggerating either)

Life-Changing

There are thousands of success stories all saying the same thing: lives are changing. It has changed my life as well as my sister's and mother's. I started my fitness journey on the typical bodybuilding protocol of whey protein, chicken breasts, sandwiches and no-xpldode-crap supplements. I thought I was eating mostly *healthy* but had no clue the damage I was doing to my health. It's what the magazines like Men's Health said to do. Why would I question their recommendations? Most people in the gym were doing the same exact things as well. Finding Paleo was like being saved.

Before Paleo, I struggled hard in pursuit of my goals. I couldn't rid the fat around my midsection and love handles. It was very frustrating to train in the gym for 3 or 4 hours a day and still not reach that ripped/six-pack look I was training for. I can tell you with absolute certainty that the Paleo way of eating is the answer to the question: **What is the human diet?** We are made to eat natural food that is unprocessed. Period. It has changed my life and I know it will change yours as well.

If you want to be ripped, improve your blood lipid profile, and feel and look better, than you must go as-Paleo-as-possible. I believe in it with every ounce of my being. It will change your life. A bit Paleo is better than zero-Paleo, so don't fall into that 'all or nothing' mindset. You don't have to go strict 100%-perfect Paleo to produce life-changing results. So don't think like that.

If you fall 'off the wagon' just get right back on

The more you eat Paleo the better you will be, while the less Paleo you eat, the worse you will be. The key is to keep improving. You won't reach perfection and that's fine. Just keep improving and eventually you will reach a place where you have excellent health, a sexy-fit body, and a bright future. Crazy what a little food can do, ey?

Get Started Today!

I hope this will motivate you to start making changes in your diet. You don't have to go "all out" to benefit from eating *more Paleo*. The more you do, the more results will show.

Here are some great ways to start:

- Raid your pantry and throw away the processed crap (pasta, grains, bread, cookies, etc.)

- Say 'NO' to bread when eating out

- Stick with chicken, fish, steak, pork dishes for your entree

- Stop drinking sugar-filled drinks (including artificial sweetened drinks)

With each small change you make, you will see a small change in your body. The hardest part is getting started. Remember to take it slow, be patient, and improve your food decisions every chance you get. Each smart decision you make will repay you dividends in the future. Just as every bad decision you make will have a negative consequence later on.

Go as-Paleo-as-possible and you can reap the benefits of health, longevity, sexiness, and that good feeling of knowing you are doing something better for yourself and the world. There is nothing better!

50 Ways Improve Your Training

Not much to explain here. Just read the list and pick tips that resonate with you. Then implement them and get better.

1. **Gear up.** Get Oly shoes, some inov-8s or nano's, a speed rope, some wrist wraps, and some comfortable workout clothes.

2. **Lift heavy weights regularly.** Don't just stay in comfortable 70% zones. Push your limit... which leads perfectly to 3...

3. **Use a spotter and FAIL.** If you aren't missing reps, you aren't training hard enough. Period.

4. **Work mobility A LOT.** Before, After, During

5. **Take your training seriously**. Always strive to become better.

6. **Don't take your training too seriously.** Give yourself a break.

7. **Train with others.** It's just better.

8. **Show up no matter what.** If you aren't in the mood, here's what you do. First: Walk to your car and drive to the Box. Second: Figure the rest out later.

9. **Fast before you train.** The idea that we "need" to consume calories before, during, or after training is bullshit hype pushed on us from the bodybuilding and supplement industries. When you switch your metabolism over to training without food, you will PR more often and feel better in general. And you'll want to send me a thank you card... you're welcome.

10. Don't throw your barbell or other equipment. It's just douchey.

11. Warm-up A LOT. Make sure you focus your warm-ups and always practice proper dynamic warm-ups before you train. This will improve your results and prevent injury.

12. Motivate other athletes. To receive, you must give.

13. Practice handstands often. You have to get upside down if you want to improve them.

14. For Females (and guys who don't have strict pull-ups yet): Have someone spot your ankles as you perform strict pull-ups (push off the spotters hands to assist reps and go for failure). This is the best way to develop the dead hang pull-up that I have found.

15. Don't cherry pick your WOD's or days. Show up those days that make you want to hide. These are the days you should never skip.

16. Train your weaknesses. Really try to destroy them. This is the only way to become a better athlete in my professional opinion.

17. Utilize your coaches before and after class. They love to talk training, food, and lifestyle. Ask them questions and then shut up and listen. You will learn a LOT.

18. Ask other athletes for tips and tricks. We are all on different paths in this journey and have learned different things along the way. You never know whom you can learn from.

19. Buy a jump rope and size it to you. Then never leave it at the gym.

20. Practice double-unders every day.

21. Do a few strict pull-ups every day.

22. Do a few one-arm push-ups every day.

23. Meditate 5 minutes every day. This can improve your entire life (and your training).

24. Practice your Olympic weightlifting every day with a dowel and empty barbell. The gains you will make doing this are insane.

25. If there is an exercise you are not good at do the following: perform 3 sets of 10 as part of your warm-up every day.

26. Work on heavy, light, and moderately weighted squats every week. Doing lots of squats will produce big gains for men and women. Squats are king.

27. Practice jumping in all modalities. Over, under, on top of, sideways, backwards, long, short, high.

28. Make sure you have a very good rack position. The barbell should be completely supported by your shoulders and not your hands.

29. Train planks often. And I really mean train them. The results from these come 30 seconds after your arms start shaking. You need some mental toughness for these.

30. Learn to bounce out of the bottom of a squat. For those that have tight hips this can be difficult and that is why you should practice often with a dowel and empty barbell.

31. Do pistols at least once a week. The more the better.

32. Make sure to hit all the major lifts at least once a week. Squat, Deadlift, Press, Bench, Snatch, Clean, Jerk

33. Have a recovery plan: hot/cold water, massage, foam rolling, nutrition, ice, Epsom salt, etc.

34. Get your family involved. Who cares if you come off annoying at first? They are your family and you don't want to bury them, do you? If you really love your family, you should give a shit if they are killing themselves with shitty food and bad lifestyle habits. Start working on them NOW.

35. Do shoulder dislocates with a dowel every workout. Don't force them. Move smoothly.

36. Turn the wrists out at the bottom of the muscle-up. This will ensure you reach full extension of the elbows, lats, and shoulders.

37. Do lots of strict dips and negative holds on the rings.

38. Incorporate strongman work into your program. Sled work and the prowler can do amazing things. Walk with a sled attached to your hips (exercise credit: Louie Simmons).

39. Practice heavy farmer carries.

40. Throw things. We've been throwing spears and javelins for thousands of years.

41. Wake up to 20 push-ups every morning.

42. Do 30 air squats and 20 push-ups after every meal. This is an awesome recommendation from Tim Ferris in the 4-Hour Body and I use it all the time. It's even better after big meals.

43. Walk after every meal. This improves digestion, prevents fat gain, and makes you feel less bloated and lethargic.

44. Do travel or home WOD's if you can't make it to the gym. Check out TrainingBox.TV for free functional home fitness.

45. Practice L-sits often. Same with frog stands. These basic gymnastic skills are easy and low-stress movements that can help you become fitter.

46. Listen to your coaches! They see what you don't see and they know their shit.

47. Work on your lifestyle and nutrition. Check out MarksDailyApple.com for more help with this.

48. Take REST days. I know it's an insane concept, but you CAN'T train every single day. High-intensity training is very stressful on your body and requires adequate rest. If you want to live a long life, and give your body the time to get stronger, you must let it repair itself through proper rest and recovery.

49. Take a REST week every couple months. This has done wonders for a lot of my athletes.

50. The best thing you can do when training is LISTEN TO YOUR BODY. You must learn when you can push past your redline and when it's time to back off. Listen to your body when it tells you to rest. Figure out what your body responds to and what it doesn't. Self-experimenting allows you to develop a plan that works for your goals and body type.

Why You Don't Have Abs (it's your food dummy)

Training Hard And Not Eating Well

I see the following quite often:

- •Athletes work their ass off in the gym (some every day)

- •They get stronger and fitter

- •But they never reach the body results they SHOULD

My box— The Training Box —has over 350+ athletes. I have observed many of these athletes train a multiple days a week for long periods of time. What I see much more than I would like to are plateaus. And it's always the same body-comp culprits: lack of sleep, drinking too much, and a shitty diet. Diet comprises approximately 80% of what determines your body composition and health (granted you aren't doing crack or smoking cigarettes).

People will usually listen when you give them nutrition advice, but very few of them will ever act on that advice. There are many factors why this is so: confusion, false food beliefs, not actually caring, not knowing where to start, skepticism, etc.

In my experience, it usually boils down to two types of athletes:

- •Clients who seek answers, absorb information, and make changes

- •Everyone else

This chapter is for the *everyone else*. I want to motivate you, nudge you, or scare you into taking action: small action, large action, any action. I want you to understand how important your food choices are. I want every bite, sip, or nibble of your favorite junk food to elicit a pang of guilt. Then, with enough guilt and knowledge, you might start making the change.

Mindset is Everything

If you can start viewing your food through new eyes, you can start making real changes. It's all rooted in your belief system. Start thinking of food as a drug. Just like a drug, it should be consumed in moderation. If you take too much of a drug, you will overdose. Like any pill, your food should contain a warning and dosage label. Drugs and food both stimulate a hormonal response in the body. For better or worse, hormones control everything in our lives:

- Happiness

- Depression

- Motivation

- Energy

- Sex drive

- Weight loss

- Weight gain

- Anger

- Stress

Do you see how food could be pretty damn important? This list comprises just about everything you do in your life and your hormones are at the root of them all. Your food can improve your life or take away from it. It's as simple as that.

Food is Everything

We all want to look better, that's a given, right? Well, I'm going to let you in on a little secret grasshopper; you ready for this? **Food determines your body**. I don't care if you have amazing genetics and can look ripped on a cupcake diet, you **will** pay for your poor food choices one way or another. Sure, you hear stories of NFL stars eating fried chicken all day and performing like machines. They are the exception, not the rule. Plus, being jacked doesn't mean you are healthy anyways. Your body is a machine that requires a certain level of maintenance, fuel, and loving care. And just like a machine, if you abuse it or neglect its maintenance, it will break down and end up in the junkyard (aka graveyard).

We all know the type that seems to have the 'skinny gene' and eat junk food like it's going out of fashion. Well, unfortunately for them, they are destroying their bodies and promoting cancer and disease and it's going to catch up to them eventually. Think back to those girls that were perfect in high school. We all know the type. I bet you can go on Facebook right now and find that many of them are now overweight. That is a diet that didn't adapt to match an aging and deteriorating body. Your body eventually breaks down from misuse; it's inevitable.

You are what you eat. You've heard this a thousand times, so why then are you still eating goddamn pop tarts? You want your ass or stomach to look and feel like gooey cherry-red filling? [Face Palm. The frustration of being a Coach in this business.]

Colin's "Three Food Rules"

1. Eat Real Food

- It shouldn't include chemicals or synthetic alterations

- It shouldn't last weeks, months, or years

- It should be prepared well and respected

- It should have been alive recently

- It should be unprocessed

- It should go bad if it sits on the counter

What this looks like: Animals, Seafood, Tubers, Sweet Taters, Veggies, Fruits, Nuts, Seeds, Pastured/Grass-Fed dairy products

What this doesn't look like: Grains, Beans, Lentils, Bread, Processed sweets, cookies, cake, juice, soda, artificial sweeteners, margarine, seed oils, refined sugar/salt

2. Cook something damn it

If you want to control what food you are eating (and you freaking should) then you need to do most of your eating at home where you have the control. Restaurants use cheap crap ingredients to save on food costs. They inflate meals with unnecessary calories and junk to make the food taste better and become more addictive (sugar, salt, msg, etc.). Listen, I'm not demonizing all restaurant food. I love to eat out, but it's best to choose places that serve local ingredients and focus on the food quality because the fact is: <u>most restaurants suck and most eating-out food is extremely unhealthy</u>.

Restaurant food:

- **Pros:** Relatively quick (depends), no clean up or prep

•**Cons:** expensive, processed, terrible for you, makes you gassy, makes you fat

Home cooked food:

•**Pros:** Cost effective, healthy, clean/unprocessed, tastes way better if done right, the key to a six-pack

•**Cons:** Shopping, clean up, prep

Reaching a high level in anything requires consistent action steps. The key is turning these steps into habits and staying consistent with them long enough to reach your goals. You want to build these habits into your being so that they are a part of who you are and what you do—they should become part of your identity.

With enough effort, you will eventually build a lifestyle, health, and body that you are proud of. Because food is 80% or more of the entire equation, this is where we start. *Never underestimate its importance.*

3. Utilize Slow Cooking

A complaint I hear often about eating clean is the amount of time it takes and I do agree with this to an extent. This is why we must use techniques like slow cooking, batch cooking, and leftover saving to make our diet easier to maintain. With any new endeavor, simplicity is king. You want to focus on getting food to your table the easiest way possible.

Enter slow cooking. Slow cooking is easy, can produce amazing meals, and requires minimal shopping, prep, and clean up. Buy a slow cooker and start using it today. It may be the missing ingredient in your food program. This single tool can change your life.

Let's Review

1. Eat Real Food
2. Cook something damn it
3. Utilize slow cooking

Don't fall into the trap of thinking you have to go *all or nothing*. It all starts with one step: one change, one habit, one meal, one dish, one anything.

"The journey of a thousand miles begins with a single step"

-Chinese proverb

Start making changes immediately:

- Eat out less
- Start cooking more
- Slow cook ONE MEAL (and then another and another)
- Skip dessert one time, two times, etc.

No one develops a new habit overnight. It takes time, and sometimes a lot of it. What I need you to do is get the importance of food imprinted on your brain. If you can truly understand how important the food you eat is for your health and results, you'll start making better decisions on a regular basis. After that, as your food decisions get better and better, your results will start to creep in. This is what I want for you.

Don't procrastinate: you either start today or you never will. Telling yourself that you will start your diet tomorrow is nonsense; you are lying to yourself. There is no tomorrow, next year, or later.

There is only now.

Get your ass in gear and make your food important **now** and **forever**.

The Trinity

For most of us, it's impossible to know exactly where our ideas come from. Our beliefs have been shaped by our experiences over the years, with most of it happening behind the scenes that is our subconscious. The thing about our beliefs is, once they take hold, it is extremely difficult to change them. It takes a massive amount of effort to overcome the beliefs and biases we have developed our entire lives. To further compound the issue, humans have a handy psychological trick that we use to delude ourselves into believing what we want. The mind tricks us into believing things that don't always reflect what is best for us. This is known as cognitive bias.

According to Wikipedia, *cognitive bias* is defined as:

A cognitive bias is a pattern of deviation in judgment, whereby inferences of other people and situations may be drawn in an illogical fashion. Individuals create their own "subjective social reality" from their perception of the input. An individual's construction of social reality, not the objective input, may dictate their behavior in the social world. ***Thus, cognitive biases may sometimes lead to perceptual distortion, inaccurate judgment, illogical interpretation, or what is broadly called irrationality.***

Some cognitive biases are presumably adaptive. Cognitive biases may lead to more effective actions in a given context. Furthermore, cognitive biases enable faster decisions when timeliness is more valuable than accuracy, as illustrated in heuristics. Other cognitive biases are a "by-product" of human processing limitations, resulting from a lack of appropriate mental mechanisms, or simply from a limited capacity for information processing.

A continually evolving list of cognitive biases has been identified over the last six decades of research on human judgment and decision-making in cognitive science, social psychology, and behavioral economics.

In short, we believe what we want to believe. Our brain will convince us of what we should believe, and sometimes in the face of overwhelming evidence to contrary. Our brain is resolute when it decides to believe something, it's a defensive mechanism. It's why we are afraid of the unknown, of different, of the eccentric. This is also why religion, politics, food, and health are so heavily debated; people have strong beliefs and their minds will do anything to hold on to those beliefs. Sometimes our beliefs are deep-rooted having developed since childhood while others are less solidified and more open to change.

Obsession

I see something all the time in my business: training turning into obsession. Many of the athletes that train high volume on a daily basis would have to look up the term "rest day" in the dictionary if asked. Some do this because they are obsessed to reach a goal, while some do it to fulfill a psychological need. No matter the reason, the fact always remains true: Without adequate recovery, there will be too much physical stress placed on the body and it will result in overtraining.

Overtraining will steal years from your life. It will ruin your joints (especially running on hard surfaces) and isn't sustainable no matter how hard you try to force it. Sure, genetics and recovery will help increase what is considered safe volume, but most go beyond what is safe on top of failing to utilize proper rest and nutrition protocols. This is a big problem.

On top of having a genuine concern for my clients and their long-term health—more than they do sometimes—I often get frustrated when they tell me about the goals they are trying to reach. Usually it's something like, "I want to lose this last 5 pounds" or "I want to lose the fat on my arms" or "I want to get rid of my love handles." And what do they do? They train more, harder, and longer. They believe that it takes more exercise to 'burn' away that last bit of fat or to 'build' that last bit of muscle. This is good intention and bad implementation, and on matter what I say they still have the belief in their mind that this is the path to take.

What they fail to realize is that training is a stress to the body. Typically, the stubborn goals that they are failing to reach are an indicator of the very stress that their overtraining is creating. Since more training is why they can't reach their goals, they should be doing less, not more. Yet more is what most of them do because they don't understand the balance between work and rest (or listen to their coach). This is the "more is better" syndrome in full effect.

This is the problem

A problem I have seen in clients over the years is they will usually seek out advice they want to hear. And when something challenges their current belief system, they will look for reasons to delude themselves into maintain their current beliefs. Furthermore, when an athlete doesn't fully understand a recommendation, or if it is too new to them, they will usually ignore it just the same.

What can we learn here? This: You must fully believe in a recommendation for it to have a real effect (and you should listen to the experts even if it's something you don't want to hear). Your subconscious is too powerful to let you do something it doesn't agree with or doesn't understand. Keep this in mind next time you pay for advice or buy that new shinny supplement. BELIEVE that it is going to work and you are a million times more likely to have it work for you. If you are at all skeptical, it won't work. This is the power of the mind. You either get it in your corner or it will fight you every step of the way.

Ready for the truth?

Be careful, what you are about to read could change your life:

MORE IS NOT BETTER. IN FACT, IT'S OFTEN WORSE!

It's important you understand what I just said to you. It's imperative that you *get* what you are reading. I will use any means to get it pounded into your head.

Examples of less is more include:

- Lifting more weight doesn't always build more muscle.

- Doing more reps doesn't always equate to increased performance.

- Running more doesn't exactly help you 'burn' more calories.

- Eating more—especially protein—doesn't magically build muscle (as the bodybuilding magazines would have you believe).

Your body is a fine balance between just enough and too much. Things that you think will get you there utilized in the wrong doses can actually screw shit up more than you can imagine. If fitness, food, health, and all of this crazy hum an-body stuff were easy, than everyone would have it figured out and a sexy bod wouldn't be so special. But it isn't easy, and most people don't have the results they want.

The Minimum Effective Dose

There is something known as the Minimum Effective Dose (MED for short). The MED is the least amount of stimuli needed to produce a desired outcome. The MED theory asserts that just enough input should be used to reach a desired result and no more. It also states that *more* often has a negative effect and the minimum should be enough for the sake of saving resources such as time, energy, and so on.

While it is difficult to find the MED without having trained for years, you can start making a conscious effort to notice what your MED is when training. As you become more conscious, and develop the awareness needed, you will become more aware of what your body is telling you. You can train harder when you do train, and rest more deliberately when you rest. You will better avoid overtraining as well as have the wherewithal to know when you need to suck it up and bust your ass. Anyone who is training to reach a goal should be conscious of the minimum effective dose. Doing so will keep you healthier, show results quicker, and allow you to enjoy your training more so.

The effect of more is exactly like the effect of less, just on the opposite end of the spectrum. At both ends you are negating your results. If you miss a month of training, your results will start sliding backwards. If you train 7 days with no rest, your results will slide backwards. We all understand that if we don't train we won't get results, right? But what about the correlation to training more and negating results? This is a less common idea because the effects aren't as apparent. With the growing popularity of HIIT training, overtraining and rest/work balance is a real concern that doesn't get the attention it deserves. Overtraining is a real thing, folks. Watch out for it. It can really screw your health and results.

Food, Sleep, Stress: The Trinity

The Trinity is: food, sleep, and stress in each of their respective manifestations. Your body is the balance of the many factors that comprise these three little words. The Trinity represents the foundation of these factors. You can't neglect any part of the Trinity and expect to reach peak body composition. If you do too much or too little in any one category, you will pay for it in health and results.

The Trinity is reflected in the habits you do on a daily basis. It is an expression of any action you take or fail to take. Act lazy and you will become weaker. Neglect sleep and you will be tired and weaker. Become more active and you will become fitter. Lift weights and you will become stronger. And so on. While you might understand this simple illustration, you probably don't fully understand just how important the balance of the Trinity is. The Trinity is non-negotiable. You must respect its importance.

What you can do is focus on improving your weaknesses as they relate to The Trinity. Instead of doing more of what you are good at—training for example—you should focus on the things you aren't good at like your diet, your sleep, or whatever else you suck at within the Trinity. It's imperative that you remember this: **focus on the things you suck at**.

Food: You have to eat the right foods in the right amounts. Too much food and you gain body fat. Too little food and you don't supply your body with the proper fuel and nutrients for it to repair. The wrong foods in any quantity and you fuck it all up, no chance whatsoever.

Sleep: Missing out on sleep is like trying to run with your laces tied: you may get there eventually, but it's going to be a bitch and you are making it much, much, much, much harder on yourself. Your body wants to win; it wants to be fit and sexy. But it **ABSOLUTELY** needs sleep. Some people get there without sleep but they are destroying their health in the process. We all love sleep and there is a reason for that. Nature has programmed us to love sleep because it is necessary for our survival, just like food. Eight Hours a night is the standard but you may need more or less. I'm not a sleep expert so look to the research for recommendations.

Stress: Stress is a bitch. It's the most under appreciated aspect of the human condition. People act like chronic stress is normal, like it's just a part of life. They don't put effort into controlling it. We are often blind to the effects of stress because we have been living with it for so many years, most of us our entire lives. It's why most of us do things to seek pleasure—so we can get relief from the fatigue of stress. Humans are not psychologically equipped to deal with the chronic mental stress that is inherent in our modern societies. The large part of our ancestral history was lived in the wild as hunter-gatherers in which we dealt with stress mostly in short bouts—like running from a predator, for example. Since the advent of agriculture and condensed population dwellings, human beings have become more stressed and fat and weak as a result.

Training is a stress. Too much stress makes you fat. Thus, too much training makes you fat (it really does). Notice I use the words "too much." On the flip side, stress also makes you stronger when applied strategically in the correct doses and balanced out with a healthy lifestyle. Most gym goers induce extreme physical stress to their bodies before hoping right back into a life filled with psychological stress. **There is no balance.** It is just stress on top of stress.

Our brains and bodies are made to deal with short bouts of stress as was necessary to survive in the wild (sprinting from a predator or after prey). We are programmed to deal with little to no access to food for periods of time, in the form of fasting. We are made to walk a lot. The average hunter-gatherer would walk about 12 miles a day while gathering, hunting, or forging for food. We are made to climb, crawl, jump, balance, and hang as is necessary in a wilderness setting. We were not made to worry about bills, pending deadlines, and constant mental stimulation via technology. This constant chatter creates mountains of stress.

Our minds have become constantly clouded with noise and distraction, much of which we don't even realize is there. We've become numb to it. We grew up with it. So how do we cope? We ignore things that are painful and use pleasure to mask the deep-rooted issues that are subconsciously dictating our lives. These ignored issues come out in the form of mind-life crises, depression, anxiety, and other clinical mental disorders. And chronic stress is at the forefront of these problems.

Stress, mental and physical, is another responsibility that requires your attention. You must be vigilant in doing things to mitigate stress. The gym is a useful stress, but what about your mental stress? Are you doing anything to reduce it? Meditation, mindfulness, taking a break, and other mental techniques can pay huge dividends.

I notice that when I am more conscious of my mental state, and practicing these concepts, my stress levels are wayyyy lower. It is too important to ignore. Try to become more conscious of your thoughts. Quiet your mind. Become aware of the present. Start addressing the nagging stress that is running your life.

Adjust The Scale

Nature is a balance—yin and yang, night and day—and so is your body. You must create a balance that will increase performance, preserve health, and enable longevity. I admit that it's not the easiest thing to do. It may take years to find the correct balance for you. It's also crazy difficult to build the many habits that are necessary to maintain The Trinity. And still, once you find the right balance, you still have to maintain it on a daily basis.

> *"The path of least resistance leads to crooked rivers and crooked men."*
> -Henry David Thoreau.

Think of each part of the Trinity as a sliding scale of one to ten. One is the least compliant and ten is the most compliant. Your goal is to strive for the best compliance (10) in EACH category. If your training and diet are a 10, but your stress is a 1 (lots of stress), you will not reach optimal results, and vice versa. Over the years, I have noticed that the best results come for people that put an equal amount into each category. You would be better served if you reached a 5-5-5 in each category over an imbalanced 9-9-1 or similarly skewed ratio.

Back to Beliefs

Your compliance to these principles is going to correlate to your beliefs. If you believe more is better, you will never be able to do less (as you should) because your subconscious will sabotage you every time. You have to believe in these concepts. You have to believe in how you train, how you eat, and how you live.

Confusion of these subjects within The Trinity is why there is so much money in the food, health, and fitness industries. There is profit in your confusion. There is a big gap between what works and what doesn't and consumers are tricked into believing the wrong shit so they will spend money on products they don't need.

As I harp on often, it's insanely difficult to change your beliefs. You aren't going to change how you think only based on what I'm writing here—hopefully it will be the start, though. Most of us brush off the things we don't want to hear. Try to catch yourself doing this. Try to be conscious of your subconscious beliefs. Through effort and awareness, you can eventually squash the limiting beliefs that are holding you back. The best way to find the truth is to read, ask questions, and seek answers to anything that confuses you. Knowledge is power as it pertains to your belief system. The stubborn minded are ignorant because they don't allow themselves to learn.

To learn is to challenge your beliefs; it is an affront to the ego. Do it as much as possible.

The ego wants to believe what it believes. It must maintain the status quo. If you want to reach physical and mental enlightenment, you need to drop that ego crap right now. You need to be open-minded and learn anyway you can, from anyone you can. I am not pretending to have all the answers. I use what works for me, what I have seen work with thousands of people, and what solid research suggests. Learn what you can from me and then go elsewhere to learn even more. Utilize as many sources of knowledge as possible.

Now that we have covered mindset, and I assume you understand how important it is, it's time to review specific recommendations for The Trinity. These recommendations are general guidelines and should be tweaked to your preference. Some may respond differently than others. Some may need to do slightly more or slightly less (or a lot more or a lot less). Keep that in mind with any recommendation:

you must always find your style. Because you are a unique individual, specific recommendations or programs may not always completely work for you as prescribed. As a result, you may need slight iterations to find what works for you. Always be testing and tweaking.

The Foundation

The Foundation is the general template for those looking to lose weight and be healthy. It encompasses the basics of what makes a human healthy. No matter your goal, you should follow this template as a baseline. You can pursue specific goals *after* you build the foundation.

Stress

The stress category includes any stress, good or bad. This encompasses reduction of stress as well as planned doses of beneficial stress.

Training:

> •4 Days a week of training (3 is the sweet spot)(high intensity WODs/strength training, etc.)
>
> •2 days should be full rest (move, walk a lot, etc.)
>
> •1 day should be active recovery (can be yoga, mobility work, skill session, etc.)

Sleep:

- Sleep 8 hours a night or more.

- Sleep in a dark room with no electronics or artificial light.

- Wake when your body tells you to.

- Find your average to feel great. I have to sleep 7 hours every night or I feel like liquid death. If you are the type of person that can sleep 10+ hours a night if you let yourself, you might be chronically sleep deprived.

Lifestyle:

•Walk every day as much as possible.

•Maintain social relationships.

•Smile, laugh, play games, and have fun as often as possible.

•Meditate as often as possible (5 minutes a day can be life changing).

•Be in the now, be present. Quiet your mind.

•Slow down. Stop that rushed, nagging, worrying mindset.

•Don't road rage. Be conscious of it and ignore it.

•Read a lot. Reading is training for your mind. Recommended subjects: Stoicism, philosophy, and psychology.

Food:

•2-3 meals a day max, no snacking.

•Protein and fat as the focus of your meals (best quality possible, Kerrygold butter, coconut oil, fatty wild caught fish, grass-fed animals).

•Yams, nuts/seeds, veggies, some fruit to fill out the rest.

•Aim for an 8-hour feeding window followed by a 16-hour fasting window every day/night.

•Eat an unprocessed Paleo/Primal diet consisting of the best foods possible from the best sources.

Common Body Types and Goals

Gain Muscle:

•Eat lots of clean animal proteins and healthy fats (Coconut oil, Grass-fed butter).

•Utilize IF with an 8-hour feeding window followed by a 16-hour fast.

•Have the biggest meal of the day immediately after you train. Load up with starchy carbs via sweet potatoes and veggies.

•Take ZMA or a magnesium supplement.

•Eat slow and eat a reasonable amount of calories.

•Lift heavy weight with as many sets as possible in the 5-10 rep range. More sets AND more weight.

•Use the following accessory movements: weighted dips, pull-ups, push-ups, jerks, cleans, and presses.

Lose Body fat:

• Utilize IF with an 8-hour feeding window followed by a 16-hour fast.

•Eat lots of clean fats and moderate protein.

•Avoid sugar at all cost.

•Consume fewer carbs, less than 100g a day.

•Walk a ton, especially after meals.

•Take 5g of fish oil a day.

•Do anything and everything to reduce stress (this is right behind your diet in importance).

•Sleep 8 hours a night - no exceptions.

•Don't beat yourself down too much in the gym. Less is more until you get lean and fit.

"Tone" (I hate that word):

•Follow the foundation and the "lose body fat" recommendations

•Lift heavy weights

•Supplement your heavy sets with lots of 10-20 rep accessory movements

•Sprint once a week

Gain weight (hard gainers):

•Eat a ton of calories

•Follow the foundation recommendations

•Eat a ton of calories

•Make mega shakes of fat, protein, and carbs

•Eat a ton of calories

•Eat a ton of calories

Get ripped:

•Eat as clean as possible

•Get on a supplement program: Vitamin D, Fish Oil, Magnesium/ZMA, digestive enzyme, green tea, black coffee

•Eat slow

•Utilize IF with an 8-hour feeding window followed by a 16-hour fast

Body Types Recommendations

Stubborn body fat on an already lean/strong physique:

•You are doing too much and the stubborn fat stores are from stress. They will NEVER go away no matter how hard you train

•Train less and spend more time on recovery

•Sleep should be of paramount importance

•Cut out shakes, bars, or other quick-digesting snack type foods

•Watch your sugar intake and stay low carb

Too skinny:

•Eat more freaking calories

•Especially protein and fat

•Consider doing less steady-state cardio

•Endurance training should be cut down

•Go for short-fast-hard sessions and lots of weight lifting

•Utilize protein shakes of fat and protein if you have trouble consuming enough calories

Big/strong but no abs:

•Watch sugar intake

- Watch calorie consumption when you do eat (these often overeat)

- Eat slow

- Walk everyday

- Avoid shakes and eat whole food

Closing

Focus on The Trinity. This is going to be enough for 95% of you. Most of you are lacking in multiple categories. The closer to 10 you get on the compliance scale, the closer you will get to your goals. It's that simple and that powerful. If you are already strong in one category, yet weak in another, than you know **exactly** what you need to focus your time on. Get in there and do the work.

The most difficult part of the trinity is mental stress in my opinion (it could be different for you). Most of us are blind to our subconscious. The simple act of thinking about thinking can do wonders. The next time you get angry, remind yourself that you are angry. Remind yourself that your anger is making you fat.

Remember, a spike in your emotions is a spike in your hormones. A spike in your hormones is bad because it causes fat gain and destroys muscle mass. Besides, angry people are weak minded and pathetic. The truly strong have control of their emotions and bodies. They are in control of their food, sleep, and stress. They are in control of The Trinity.

"Strong people are harder to kill and more useful in general"

-Mark Rippetoe.

OMG it's Gluten-Free...

The food(s) that is killing you.

It all started with *low-fat*. The low-fat marketing campaign was an early player in the processed food revolution known as *Operation Make America Fat and Sick*. Let's look at how it all got started.

What happens when I say the word fat? What is the first image that pops in your head? You probably visualize an obese man or women or maybe Jabba the Hutt if you are a Star Wars fan. Regardless of what visuals appear in your head, it's almost universal in this country that the word fat has is linked to being overweight. When we hear that someone is 'fat' we think of an abundance of adipose tissue—or the more politically correct vernacular, being obese.

No one wants to be fat, right? Well than, it would *seem* intuitive to give people the following advice: "Don't eat fat because it makes you fat." Sure, that makes sense and I could see how it could become a popular notion. Unfortunately, the common sense of the masses is almost always wrong. And there is no better evidence of this than the ideas surrounding fat, cholesterol and what is considered a "healthy" diet. The idea that fat is going to make you fat, or eating cholesterol is going to clog your arteries, are two of the most health destroying ideas ever introduced to the American people.

America, The Land of The... Fat People?

It's easy to dupe a large number of people with any common-sense-sounding assertion if it is passed around enough. The government and politicians have been utilizing this psychological trick for years. All you need to do is *loosely* (sometimes very loosely) connect the dots in a way that seems to make sense and the human yearning to believe will kick into full-effect. Little research or question will go beyond initial statements, and before you know it, something someone said on TV is now "common knowledge." When this happens, the people that try to refute it are just brushed off and labeled something that makes it easy to ignore them, such as paranoid, tin-foil hat wearer, bias, etc. The reason is the average person doesn't want to think. It wants to be told what is what. It wants absolutes. People want the easy way and they will believe whatever everyone else believes because it's easier (see the concept "Mob mentality").

Somehow triglycerides, which are an essential macronutrient and building block of life, become know as fats—I'm not familiar with how this happened but that's neither here nor there. Vilifying fat by correlating dietary fat with being physically fat created the opportunity for food companies to initiate the processed food campaign. This created the low-fat label that ended up becoming one of the most detrimental marketing campaigns in U.S. history (second only to the "American Dream" by Fanne and Freddy). Low-fat swept the nation like wildfire with the help of faulty research from Ancel Keys and the *Lipid Hypothesis*. This helped spit out evil offspring in the form of the *low cholesterol* and the *heart healthy* nonsense promoted by the American Heart Association (think Cheerios).

The Accidental Conspiracy That Is Now Probably A Conspiracy

This accidental conspiracy was birthed from an opportunity made possible by a combination of faulty research, government regulation, and corporate greed. It grew the cheap-food-monster into a multi-billion dollar a year industry. And then came the final piece to this already massive harbinger-of-death consortium: the pharmaceutical companies.

In came drugs, the legal kind. People got sick form the shitty food and they went to their doctors for help. Drugs were created to fulfill the demand; lots of money to be captured, huge markets created, huge demand to fill. The food industry fueled the drug industry's growth to massive proportions (I personally think it's the main reason).

The cycle goes like this:

1. Eat cheap, processed food based on recommendations from faulty research and marketing claims.

2. Gain weight, ruin your metabolism, throw your hormones out of whack, and completely mess yourself up.

3. Go to the doctor and get pills to maintain your symptoms (Band-Aid). Keep the same diet and lifestyle habits. Become a customer for life. Eventually seek more medication as your current medication loses its effectiveness. Repeat this process until you find yourself on a handful of medications with your health slowly slipping away.

A Big Fat Conspiracy of Government Regulation, Food Companies, And Drug Companies

These "big three" are responsible for destroying this country's health. There's really no other way to put it. I call it an accidental conspiracy because it wasn't planned, it just kind of happened. The science wasn't understood at the time. They just got lucky and capitalized on a new market. These conspirators unknowingly joined forces and now our country is sick and getting sicker while corporations are making billions of dollars keeping us stuck in this profitable matrix.

I want you and our future generations to escape this destructive cycle. But you will only escape if you are armed with the truth. This will allow you to start making decisions that keep you out of the cycle. Some techniques you can start immediately to reverse this trend include buying local food, supporting small family farms, and avoiding any and all products from the big food companies.

The saga continues

After low-fat came low-carb. Low-carb was a response to the low-carb Atkins and South Beach diet trends. Products were promoted as low-carb to dupe consumers into buying a product that was perceivably *healthier* for them because it was based on these new diet recommendations. ***Fooled again***. Unfortunately, what consumers ended up consuming was food that was *more* processed and *more* damaging to their health. The companies replaced the carbs with other processed ingredients and slapped a shiny new label on it.

Low-fat and low-carb are still kicking today. You will probably notice it everywhere the next time you go grocery shopping. And this brings us to the most recent trend in the food space, Gluten-Free. Gluten-free may be the most difficult of these marketing labels to dispel; it just screams *I'm better*. It is supported by the popularity of the Paleo and Primal diets and the gluten-free awareness that is sweeping the nation. Even I find myself getting sucked into this vortex of marketing bullshit from time to time. In fact, I recently realized this hard truth as I was staring at an empty box of gluten-free chocolate chip cookies (I had just eaten 1100 calories, WTF was I thinking?).

The Gluten-Free Revolution

This one is near and dear to my heart because of the gluten-free emphasis in the Paleo diet (which I endorse and eat). I know many of us are falling for the gluten-free trap and it is leading us into eating more processed foods. It's totally working for the food companies, hence the massive rise in everything having a gluten-free sticker on it.

Wait a minute, isn't gluten-free healthy?!

You aren't asking the right questions Neo...

Gluten-free is better for you than gluten filled, sure, this is true of any food product. But that doesn't mean jack when determining the food as a whole, and what ingredients make up the product. Most importantly, the majority of "gluten-free" labeled food is processed. Gluten is found in grain/wheat products and is also used as a preservative in other foods such as sauces, marinades, and dressings. These foods are bad whether they are gluten-free or not because, well, umm, **they are processed foods**!

Let's connect-the-dots in reverse on this one. You won't find gluten in the produce section. You will usually find it in the dry goods and cold food areas, though. Examples of commonly filled-with-gluten items include: store-made potato salads, sushi, wraps, pasta, sandwiches, bread, crackers, bars, soy sauce, BBQ sauces, wheat, frozen meals, etc. Products containing gluten are almost always empty calories. These processed products contain large amounts of carbohydrates and little in the way of healthy fats, protein, or vitamins and minerals. A simple way to figure out if a GF product is healthy or not it is to do a little test. **If a food is not healthy with gluten in it than it will not be healthy with gluten removed.** A processed food with gluten removed is just a more-processed food. Make sense?

This is what the low-carb and low-fat model has done since the beginning: Take something out and replace it with something else to support a label. Let's look at some examples of common gluten-free products that consumers buy:

- Gluten-Free bread

- Gluten-Free cookies

- Gluten-Free crackers

- Gluten-Free Pasta

- Gluten-Free protein bars

- Gluten-Free chips

- Gluten-Free biscuits

- Gluten-Free Pizza

Are any of these items considered healthy, gluten free or not? Of course not, this is just processed food, and when it's gluten-free, it's just more processed food. So, we can safely conclude that the majority of gluten-free-labeled foods are simply not good for you.

I want you to be weary of falling into the gluten-free trap. Especially those of you that are gluten-free, Paleo eating practitioners like myself. It's easy to get excited when we see gluten-free. It's easy to see a box of gluten-free this or gluten-free that and think DAMMMMMN there is my ticket to the good life. Then, a box of cookies later and you're in 1000 empty calories, a stomachache, and wondering WTF just happened. (Sounds like my average Wholefoods experience.)

Just Say No

I see it all the time while standing behind the poor souls in line at the register: carts full of GF-labeled crackers, cookies, pasta, and all kinds of other processed food (if you can even call it that). Don't do this. Please. Remember, *gluten-free does not mean good for you.* A processed food is still processed when the gluten is removed. Also remember, your diet should consist of whole ingredients that are direct from nature with minimal to no processing: farm direct, nature direct, local, and organic are some examples.

A disclaimer: Not all food products that sport a gluten-free label are bad. In fact, you would prefer if your food labels always said GF because this means that no gluten is added as a preservative (which you can sometimes find in sausage and other flavored meat products). What I want you to be conscious of is the trap of buying processed food that is masked as healthy via a big fat GF label. Products you prefer to see a GF label on include sausage, spice blends, protein powders, cured meats, and other Paleo-friendly, non-grain products. The GF label on certain products does help provide the peace of mind that the food is a bit closer to nature and doesn't have any added gluten-based preservatives. This is where a GF label can benefit us.

In Closing

This was originally intended as a response to all the gluten-free marketing I have been seeing lately, but now I realize the message is bigger than that. **It's about the food industry as a whole.** Don't fall into the cycle of becoming a consumer of cheap, processed food. Low-fat, low-carb, gluten-free, lactose-free, vitamin this, vitamin that, and even organic are usually just marketing labels and do not tell the whole story of where the food came from, how it was treated, and what's in it. Dig deeper and understand what you are buying, where it comes from, how it was made, and what has been added or taken away.

How to be a smart consumer:

- Be Informed

- Be a label reader

- Be a Googler of the company whose products you buy

- Buy local

- Support small farms

- Buy whole-fresh ingredients that are straight from nature

Be smart about your food choices. Buy smaller brands that put an emphasis on the ingredient, where it comes form, and the environmental implications. You will feel better about what you are eating and enjoy the better results of eating more nutritious food. It's incredible how powerful food really is.

Why should you care about the quality of your food? Simple, because you get to enjoy these benefits:

- Six-pack abs

- Lean

- Sexy

- Get stronger

- Run faster, jump higher, move better

- Live longer

- Sleep better

- Have better sex

- And everything else that comes with amazing health

Remember, food is everything when it comes to your body and health (broken record, I know).

Beware of the marketing traps, shop smarter, and eat better.

Weaknesses and Why We Suck at Not Sucking

I'm good at the snatch because I have a deep squat and enough hip mobility that allows me to get under the bar fast. I can lift well above my bodyweight. Ironically though, my back squat is my weakest lift. I'm also good at muscle-ups: I can do 30 in under 5 minutes. Ironically though, my chest doesn't grow (Grr) and it's my most underdeveloped body part. So what do I train most often? Yup, muscle-ups and snatches. Why do I do this when it makes so much sense to focus on my weaknesses?

DAMN GOOD QUESTION!

Ask yourself that same question and I bet you will end up with the same head-scratching answer. Yet, we all do it. *Why do we cherry pick so much?* Maybe it's easier. Maybe we will feel strong all the time. Maybe it's ego soothing. Maybe it is more fun. Maybe we want to be that much better so we can impress others. The list goes on. For me, it's definitely: because it hurts less.

Have you noticed—or is it only me—that when you train things you suck at it seems to hurt so badly? I haven't figured out if this is my Ego hurting or my underdeveloped muscles screaming out (probably the Ego). The irony here is if I train smarter by focusing on my weaknesses, I can improve my strengths as well. By developing my weaknesses, I see improvement in e-v-e-r-y-t-h-i-n-g. *Isn't it ironic? Don't ya think?*

As a new trainee, you need to learn fast the importance of training your weaknesses. Just getting in the gym consistently is your challenge but as time goes on and you improve, you will find yourself favoring your strengths while naturally avoiding your weaknesses. It's inevitable. Active trainees get this. We know we do it, too. Unfortunately, what we know and what we do are not always equal (ain't that the freakin truth).

This is a call to action: I want you to act, to make a change. I'm planting a seed in your mind in the hope that this idea—weakness training—will pop into your consciousness often enough to annoy the hell out of you until you do something about it. Each time you step in the gym, ask yourself this question: "Am I training a weakness?"

Progress and Tracking

They say what gets measured gets improved. I agree. I suggest you get a WOD journal, or write your workouts in a text doc on your phone. You want to get your mind to fixate on improving your numbers. Get into the constant improvement mindset.

Sure, this is a beat-to-death recommendation that has been made by every fitness guru since Richard Simmons (don't quote me on that, that may not be true). You've heard the importance of tracking your workouts a thousand times. **So, why aren't you doing about it?**

Start a workout journal, and make sure you put an emphasis on tracking your weaknesses. By tracking them, you are forced to put numbers to them: sets, reps, weight, etc. This ties something tangible to your weaknesses and it is often the missing link to the typical *"Train your weaknesses"* suggestion. By introducing numbers you see a clear path for improvement. It becomes much easier than the arbitrary "work on your weaknesses." When you have numbers, it's simple: just improve the numbers!

We all know we should train our weaknesses but how often are we training them? For most, it's not often. It's rare that we develop a plan for our weaknesses. We usually just show up at the gym and do a set here or there. Let's avoid that crap. It's time to do something about it: put it down on paper, train daily, and integrate it into your program. *If you have competition goals, weaknesses should be the focus of your training; it should be your gospel.*

Classes

What about training in a class setting? Classes can make weakness training difficult because you have to follow the programming made for everyone. You'll have to do your best to fit your weakness training in. If it conflicts with the WOD for the day, you might start looking for excuses to put it off altogether. The more you avoid training your weaknesses, the more likely it will end up another fallen habit (also known as good intention). Figure out when you will spend time training. Then do it. Commit to it.

You must make weakness training a priority. Write it down and make yourself do it. There are many ways to go about the doing, that's the easy part:

> • You could choose one day a week and completely destroy yourself using only exercises you suck at.
>
> • You could do a few deliberate sets every workout.
>
> • You could train ONLY your weaknesses every workout for a month before going back to your regular program (a basic form of periodization)

Let's look at two formats

Option 1:

Pick two main weaknesses. Mix up rep schemes, weights, and exercises but make it look something like this:

Weakness 1# for 5 sets of 15+ reps as part of your warm-up, strength, or cool down
Weakness 2# for 5 sets of 15+ reps as part of your warm-up, strength, or cool down

Lots and Lots and Lots and Lots of reps are the key here. Most weaknesses stem at the movement level where the body is weak due to flexibility, body type, past injury and so on. Tons of reps focused on super-solid form can help correct this. Start with bodyweight loads, and then progress to light, medium, and heavy loads, as you are able to. Add weight only when your form improves. Your weakness training doesn't have to infringe on your daily workout. Just treat it as a warm-up or skill work on days that it could get in the way of your program.

Option 2:

Make a list of 5-10 weakness-based exercises and do them as your warm-up as often as possible.

A warm-up (or WOD) could look something like this:

- •3 rounds of 15 reps:

- •Air Squat

- •Pistol

- •Push-up

- •Dip

- •Strict pull-up

- •Back squat with bar/dowel

- •Overhead squat with bar/dowel

You can mix this up as you see fit, but the general idea is to complete these movements each and every workout as your standard warm-up. The basic premise is the more reps you do the better you will get.

These weakness templates should be experimented with. Plus, since we live in *constantly-varied land*, you are encouraged to mix it up anyway. The beautiful thing about creating these weakness-wods is you kill two birds with one stone: you improve metabolic conditioning via high-intensity training and you improve your weaknesses by doing tons and tons of reps.

Recap

> **1. Start!** Day in, day out, workout after workout, start training your weaknesses as a pillar of your training.
> **2. Do lots and lots of reps with perfect form.** Increase weight as form improves, not before.
> **3. Track what you are doing.** This will keep you focused on what you are doing and it will allow you to know when to scale up or down.

When I think of weakness training I always remember Arnold when he talked about bodybuilders being sculptors in the movie "Pumping Iron." He said that bodybuilders think like a sculptor and if he needs more deltoids he "exercises to put those deltoids on"--like an artist adding clay to a statue. Sure, we aren't bodybuilders, but we are trying to slap improvement and development onto our bodies just the same. This quote applies perfectly to this process.

Target your weaknesses until they are no longer weaknesses.

How To Eat Clean with The Paleo Diet

The adage is true: you are what you eat. Never have truer words been uttered, and never have truer words been more ignored.

So you wanna be strong like a bull? Simple: eat grass-fed beasts, wild animals and seafood. You probably don't wanna be weak, unhealthy, and disgusting? Well, that's what you become if you eat processed foods in the form of refined grains, sugars, and other preservative-filled junk food.

Eating a Paleo diet, also known as the caveman diet or the hunter-gatherer diet, makes men and women healthy, fit, and functional. It improves every aspect of human health. Just like a cow or gorilla has a natural diet, so does a human. **Paleo is the human diet**.

It's time to forget anything you have heard about this or that diet. In fact, strike the word "diet" from your vocabulary right now. When you think of food and nutrition, think of whole, natural food—also known as "real food." Eating real food is the key to reaching the body and health you've always wanted.

It's estimated that nutrition makes up 80% of what determines your long-term health and body composition. Think about that for a second. Eighty-freaking-percent. Do you think that a bottle of pills, some protein powder, and a gym membership—which all fall into the 20% category—are going to overcome the other 80% that is proper nutrition? (This is a rhetorical question.)

Sure, I can lecture you on the merits of nutrition all day long (actually, it's a hobby of mine), but no matter what:

•I can't do your grocery shopping for you

- I can't keep you from ordering that fried chicken

- I can't stop you from eating the bread the waiter brings you at

- I can't make you fast and eat fewer meals

- I can't prevent you from drinking gluten-filled beer and sugar-filled mixed drinks every weekend

- I can't make you put down the fork

No, I can't make you do any of that. What I can do, however, is arm you with the knowledge to help you start the change that could save your life—and I'm gonna do everything I can to try convince you to help yourself.

Changing your diet is difficult. For some of you, it could be the most difficult thing you've ever done. It can take months, even years, and you will progress only a little at a time. But please, please listen to me when I tell you this:

It'll be worth every single bit of effort a hundred thousand times over!

And don't forget: anything worth having only comes after effort. If you want to reap the benefits—in this case, having a sexy bod and life-long health—than you must invest the time.

Think: Investing

Any action you take in life will always produce a result, for better or worse. If you waste one hour of your day watching mindless TV, you might lose hundreds of hours in the future from the lack of exercise and damage to your brain cells. If you spend a dollar on pointless crap today—instead of investing it—you will lose out on much more in the future by failing to invest those dollars. When it comes to food investing is the perfect analogy: **You are investing in your health on a daily basis with every thing you do (or fail to do).**

Life is a marathon. Treat it as such

You can't win a marathon by sprinting and you can't win it by going too slow. You have to stay at a moderate pace long enough to get to the finish line. If you work consistently towards your goals on a day-to-day basis, you will eventually reach them. Goals with food are just this: a marathon. Unfortunately, most don't have the endurance to keep going. They wax and wane, they yo-yo, and given enough time, they revert to old ways.

At the beginning of every New Year, gyms sell a ton of memberships to people who have convinced themselves that this year will be different. Yet, it never is. Most people last a month or two before falling back into their old habits. If your health isn't important enough to you now, it will never be important enough. I hate to sound pessimistic, especially because I am an eternal optimist, but I have seen it far too many times to spin it any other way. I truly hope that many of you can make the change and reach real results. That said, you should prepare yourself for what it's going to take. To get those results, you must commit to yourself with every fiber of your being. If you don't, you won't make it.

Personal Development

One thing I love about personal development and improving one's health and fitness is the carry-over it has to everything else in life. If you can eat a clean diet and stay on an exercise protocol, you can do *anything*. Health improvements are some of the hardest habits to maintain for humans living in our modern world; it's far too easy to give up.

I always recommend that nutrition be at the forefront of people's efforts. Making improvements in your diet will have huge carry-over to other things you are working on like training, stress, sleep, etc.

So what do I eat?

The short answer: some damn good food. With that long introduction out of the way, I will now get down to the specifics. Proper nutrition is pretty simple to understand. Don't let the newest "expert" or "guru" tell you otherwise. Many people get hung up on trying to find perfection and end up worrying about trivial things when they should be focusing on the basics:

- Food quality (buy the best you can find and afford)

- Eat meals and avoid snacking (2-3 meals a day)

- Skip meals if not hungry

- Avoid sugar, grains, lentils, beans, rice, processed food, most dairy, and all processed food

If you stay in the realm of this short list for the majority of what you do (remember, it's never about being perfect), you will achieve excellent health and body composition. You will look, feel and perform better at everything in life.

FOOD in a nutshell

Eat the highest quality meats, seafood, nuts, seeds, vegetables, fruit, and starches you can find. You should also include grass-fed butter and organic coconut. This style of eating is based on the hunter-gatherer diet that humans have survived on for thousands of years before the advent of agriculture. There are cultures that still eat this way everyday in remote parts of the world where industrialization has yet to infect. Across the board, these people enjoy excellent health that is void of heart disease, diabetes, and nearly all western disease.

Food: Where To Get It, How To Prepare It, and Restaurants Suck

Home-cooked food is ideal because you control what goes into your meals, and thus, your body. Restaurants use preservatives and processed ingredients to keep food costs low. When eating out, be picky and vocal with your server. Ask for a gluten-free menu and request butter or olive oil for cooking your meal. Typically, I tell the waiter that I have a gluten allergy and that my meal must be gluten-free. The better restaurants usually have a gluten-free menu; however, many will not. You have to ask the waiter questions and sometimes he will have to go to the kitchen and ask the chef what goes into certain dishes. **It's worth the hassle**. Try going gluten-free for 30 days then have it slip in one meal: you will bloat like the Goodyear blimp. It's not pleasant.

Home Food Prep

If you are pressed for time, or if your budget is tight, I recommend making big pot meals such as soups, stews, and braises. A crock-pot or Dutch oven is your best friend. The more you practice each of these methods, the better your dishes will get. Season each ingredient as you add it to the pot, this will develop deep flavor. Always taste throughout the cooking process and adjust with vinegar, lemon juice, salt pepper, herbs, and spices.

A basic stew/braise technique:

> 1. Preheat Dutch oven - med heat
>
> 2. Add oil
>
> 3. Sear protein on each side 2-5 minutes until crust forms
>
> 4. Remove protein
>
> 5. Add various vegetables and cook until soft and browned (onion, carrots, leeks, celery, mushrooms, potatoes, etc.)
>
> 6. Add wine or vinegar or both and deglaze pan, scraping up browned bits at bottom of pan. Return meat to pan

7. Add stock/broth/wine until fill to desired level. Optional: add tomato sauce/paste, or canned tomatoes

8. Season and bring to boil. Reduce heat and cover and cook until protein is tender 30 minutes to 2 hours depending.

9. Eat and refrigerate leftovers

The Crock-Pot method:

1. Throw in bunch of ingredients: Protein, veggies, stock, wine, vinegar, seasoning, herbs, spices

2. Cook on low 8-10 hours.

3. Serve

4. Finishing options: organic cream, garnish with herbs, chopped green onions, a splash of olive oil, or a thick-grained sea salt.

Food quality: The most important thing

Nutrition is a heavily debated topic across the Interwebz. Some people get sucked into this and end up trying to find the "answer" to nutrition. I suggest you avoid getting sucked into this rabbit-hole; it can be hard to get out of.

If you analyze hunter-gatherers that lived around the world you find completely different diets. The Inuit (Eskimos), for example, ate a diet comprised of mostly saturated fat and animal protein with little prevalence of fruits or vegetables. The Kitavans lived as islanders and consumed coconut and starchy root vegetables as the bulk of their diet with fruit and fish representing the rest of calories consumed. We find the same story as we venture around the globe and look at the diet's of people living in different geography regions; people survived on what food was prevalent in their local area. And still, what is the main thing that all of these diets have in common?

It was fresh, locally available, REAL FOOD!

The answer to nutrition is this: Eat Real Food. If you do this, you won't have any problems (actually, you'll probably change your life).

The point is to not be neurotic with your food. You don't need to read 20 books about nutrition to feel like you *have the answer*. Just Focus on eating a colorful balance of high-quality ingredients each time you sit down for a meal. That being said, everyone is different and can sustain different ratios; you just have to tweak and find your preference. My general recommendation is to eat protein and fat first—about 70-80 of your calories—and then fill out the rest with healthy, starchy carbs in the form of veggies and some fruit.

There is no one-size-fits-all answer when it comes to food ratios; this is why food quality is so damn important. 100% Paleo or not, if you consume only the highest quality ingredients, everything else tends to fall into place.

Whole foods fill you up because they are full of satisfying nutrition that signals your body that you are nourished. The same is not true of processed foods. Processed food has a reverse effect in which the body craves more calories because it isn't nourished and because processed food is usually just "empty calories." This is why processed food begets processed food. You end up eating more of the processed crap as your body craves more.

The bottom line is if you are eating a colorful diet full of fresh ingredients, and mixing it up often, it's hard to go wrong. The problem is people eat at restaurants, snack on crap, drink soda, and have other unhealthy habits that screw it all up, and worst of all, their diet is comprised mostly of processed food that comes in a package.

Meat and potatoes

A typical Paleo meal looks a lot like the *meat, potatoes, and veggies* meal that was the staple American dinner a short 30+ years ago. Unfortunately, since this time things have changed with the development of factory farming, fast food, and the low-fat food revolution. America has been convinced that eating animals is bad, that egg yolks raise your cholesterol, and that fat is the devil. What is ironic about these so-called "bad" foods is they are actually the BEST foods we can eat. If this isn't a paradox than I don't know what is.

The fat-hypothesis and other "health healthy" dogma promoted to the American public ushered in the processed food revolution and allowed corporations to produce food that was fast, easy and at the fraction of the cost. This quickly turned into a multi-billion dollar a year industry. Research done by Ancel Keys (if you can call it that) led to campaigns led by the American Heart Association and other government agencies that ended up creating the completely *inaccurate* food pyramid. I won't get into the *Meat and potatoes* (you like that?) of it right now, but I highly recommend you check out Gary Taubes book: Good Calories Bad Calories. In a nutshell: Eating cholesterol from animals is not proven to raise blood cholesterol levels nor increase the risk of heart disease (the same goes for egg yolks).

A very simple formula: eat meat, leaves, and berries. Do this and you will live a longer and more enjoyable life. Your blood lipids will improve. You will easily burn fat and build muscle. You won't feel sick, bloated, or irritated.

You can change your life with food.

Get serious about your food; make better decisions, shop local, and cook your food at home. It will change your life.

One-Pot Paleo Meals To The Busy Person's Rescue

Those who cook at home know just how extensive the process can be. Food prep, dicing, slicing, sautéing, baking, plating, eating, cleaning up, dishes, cutting board cleaning, stove cleaning, pots and pan cleaning, and so on; a freaking nightmare. When coming home from a long day of work, the last thing I want to do is go through this process from start to finish. And I bet the same goes for you.

Cooking healthy food can be a major hassle if you don't plan ahead. One of the most prevalent reasons people don't stick to their eating plan is they don't have access to food that is readily available. (My new book will help: www.GymLifeCook.com)

Food prep does take work and time, yes, we all know that, but that doesn't mean you should succumb to cheap processed food just because it is convenient. The cons far outweigh the pros when it comes to processed food.

So what are we to do? We are going to **get smart.**

Food research shows us that convenience and accessibility play a huge role in what we eat, how often we eat, and how much we eat. When food is difficult to prepare, it becomes much less likely you will eat it, and more likely to go for something else that is more convenient. This can work to your advantage by hiding sweets in hard-to-get places (or not buying altogether), or it can work against you if you have a bunch of raw ingredients in your fridge that need to be extensively prepared before being able to be eaten.

Luckily there is a solution to the problem of preparing yummy, healthy food quick and easy. It's called the One-Pot meal. This meal can be prepared in a Crockpot, Dutch oven, baking pan, or any large cooking vessel. I love the Crockpot for it's simplicity and fast clean up. You can throw a bunch of raw ingredients into the Crockpot, set it to low for 8-10 hours and bam: you have a fully cooked meal that is piping hot and ready to eat. One-Pot meals are a great "plan-ahead" way of combating the *convenience trap* that many of us fall into. Remember, clean food must be ubiquitous and easy to prepare.

Always remember that clean food must be ubiquitous and easy to prepare. On the flip side, junk food should be as inaccessible as possible. If you keep it in your house, you will eat it. If you regularly keep junk food at home (maybe for other people) then make it as difficult as possible to get to. Hide it. Forget where you put it. Tell your family to hide it. And never keep it in sight sitting on the counter.

The single most effective technique that I have found for adhering to a clean diet is making one-pot meals. I always keep a leftover meal in the fridge that can be reheated and ready to eat in minutes.

One-Pot meals...

First, buy a cast-iron Dutch oven or a Crockpot or slow cooker! My favorite brand for Dutch ovens is Staub. The goal of One-Pot meals is to make extra and save the leftovers in the fridge for future meals.

The formula for One-Pot meals = Make extra food and save the leftovers!

Certain foods keep better in the fridge than others. Stews, soups, roasts, and braises are great as leftovers and even sometimes benefit from resting in the fridge for a day or two. I suggest making 2-3 of these big meals every week with the purpose of keeping the extra in the fridge. After each pot you prepare, you will have multiple meals waiting for you in the fridge anytime you are in a rush and don't have time to cook.

There are two cooking methods for making one-pot meals that I use. Each method takes a small amount of prep work, long cooking times, and very little clean up. (Awesome, I know right!) You will need a few tools: a hand-blender or heatproof blender, Staub Dutch oven or Crockpot, a serving spoon, Sea Salt.

Method 1: Crock Pot

1. Throw in a bunch of: Protein and veggies.

2. Cover with stock, wine, and/or vinegar.

3. Flavor with: seasoning, herbs, and spices.

4. Cook on low 8-10 hours.

5. Serve.

6. Garnish options: cream, fresh herbs, splash of olive oil, sea salt, pepper, red pepper flakes, hot sauce.

Method 2: Dutch Oven

1. Preheat Dutch oven - med heat.

2. Add oil.

3. Sear protein on each side 2-5 minutes until crust forms.

4. Remove protein.

5. Add various vegetables and cook until soft and browned (onion, carrots, leeks, celery, mushrooms, potatoes, etc.).

6. Add wine or vinegar or both and deglaze pan, scraping up browned bits at bottom of pan. Return meat to pan.

7. Add stock/broth/wine until fill to desired level. Optional: add tomato sauce/paste, or canned tomatoes.

8. Season and bring to boil. Reduce heat and cover and cook until protein is tender 30 minutes to 2 hours depending on protein used.

9. Eat and refrigerate leftovers. To serve leftovers: reheat in oven at 325 for ~15 minutes or microwave on low and stir every couple minutes.

Practice Makes Yummy

The more you practice these methods, the better your dishes will get. Make sure to season each ingredient as you add it to the pot to develop that deep flavor. Taste throughout the cooking process and adjust with vinegar, lemon juice, salt, pepper, herbs, and spices.

Think of your meals as an investment in your health. Invest a couple hours each week and you will always have a quick and healthy meal in the fridge—and this can pay dividends in your health and results.

Always keep this food rule in your mind so you can use it to your advantage: The harder it is to get access to food the less likely you are to eat it. Use this to your advantage and be prepared. Now, get in the kitchen and make a one-pot meal for the upcoming week!

Create WODs and Train Anywhere

The beautiful thing about functional training is it can be done anywhere and with little to no equipment. It's possible to achieve a high level of fitness using only body-weight exercises and metabolic conditioning. While I do recommend you utilize a fundamental strength program, it is important to showcase how **easy** it is to get a workout in whether you have access to equipment or not. You should never use the gym as an excuse for not training.

Create Infinite WOD's At Home Or Travel

Below you have a simple and effective system for creating hundreds of workouts that you can do with ZERO equipment. *Never again do you have an excuse for not getting a workout in.* These workouts are perfect for traveling athletes but also serve as an excellent starting point for beginners. The only thing you ever need to do a workout is your body and the ground, and since you always have those two available, you can always get your train on. Make sense?

The 9 basic body-weight movements:

- •Push-up
- •Squat
- •Sit-up
- •Burpee
- •Lunge
- •Spring
- •Plank

•Broad Jump, Box Jump

•Handstands, Press, Kick-to, Walks, Holds,

The basic template for creating a workout that is 8-15 minutes average length is as follows:

1. Pick Total Movements (sprints, squat, etc.)

2. Pick Reps Per Movement

3. Pick Rounds or Total Reps Goal

4. Format in a repeating fashion: AMRAP (as many rounds as possible), or 1-10 rounds total, or 50-100-250 reps total, or any creative variation on these

5. Set stopwatch and go!

Example: 10 rounds of: 5 Push-ups, 5 Air Squats, 5 Sit-ups. Complete 5 push-ups, then complete 5 air squats, then complete 5 sit-ups. Repeat 10 times with proper form as fast as possible. Your score is the time that you finish (the faster the better).

Now that you have a never-ending supply of home/travel workouts, it's time to get off your ass and do some work. In as little as 15 minutes a day—or less—you can progress towards elite fitness.

That's pretty freaking awesome if you ask me.

Conclusion

Great work, you made it. *Well... not quite.*

This is just the beginning of your journey. You are now armed with some pretty snazzy knowledge that you can use to become better, but that ain't even half of the battle. You may not realize it, but you just entered a lifelong agreement with your body. It's going to be a long, often painful, journey. But that is what makes it so awesome. Savor the journey as much as the destination and when you look in the mirror at those results, you'll know what it took to get there and they will be all the more awesome.

Come back to these chapters from time to time; let them refresh you, remind you. Rereading will provide you with new ideas and insights each time. Grab a highlighter and mark lines of interest. Refer back to this highlighted text in the future and keep training your mind just as you are training your body. It's a never-ending journey.

Mental Training

Now is the time to build a life you are proud of, one that is rooted in learning and personal growth and strength. After reading this book, you should have (hopefully) opened your mind and be thinking differently, if only slightly. Keep this up. Let new ideas in. Become a seeker of the truth. Read books, articles, and blogs in pursuit of more knowledge. Accept that you, nor I, have all the answers.

And whatever you do, **be ready** because your new mindset is going to change your life. That's soooo freaking cool. I'm jealous that you get to experience this journey—it only comes once so make sure you relish it.

If you have yet to adopt this mindset, or you are hesitant, I implore you: **Do it**! It will help improve everything in your life, not just your food and fitness. Mindset dictates everything you do, for better or worse. It's about time you start getting it right. An open mind is nimble and can adapt to changes whereas a stubborn mind will lead you to a life of disappointment and constant strain.

Don't ever neglect your mental training. Your mind is a muscle, your biggest muscle, and it should be exercised as often as your body, if not more. Books are the training weights for the mind. Develop the habit of reading a little bit every day and you will be amazed by how much you'll improve. **Remember: Strengthen your mind and strengthen your body.** It all starts in your noggin. From here your actions flow. That big organ in your head is responsible for how you feel and what you do. It dictates everything.

Don't you wonder why it gets so little attention?

It's mind-boggling to me that mental development isn't more addressed in our society, especially as it pertains to tangible success. Sure, there are hundreds of self-help books that try to motivate you and incentivize you with hope and promises, but they provide little effect because they focus too much on the surface and fail to address the deep-rooted belief system that is hidden below the surface. These inner beliefs are ultimately who we are. Some are good and some are bad. The hard part is recognizing which is which, as we love to tell stories to ourselves about ourselves.

To figure out what is deep-rooted in you, you must ask yourself hard questions. You have to be honest, objective, and sometimes even get a third party opinion. This is a difficult thing to do and requires making ourselves uncomfortable. The Ego tries to protect itself at all costs; it can't stand you asking "Why." It wants to lead you blindly and keep you from calling the shots. Basically, your Ego deludes you. It keeps you blind and unaware. Your subconscious convinces your conscious mind of mistruths as a means to protect it from pain, from inquiry. Lying to yourself is real ladies and gentlemen, and most have not the slightest clue they do it.

Are you able to look yourself in the mirror and objectively ask yourself hard questions? Can you be honest with admitting your shortcomings and mistakes? Are you able to combat the bias perceptions that your Ego uses to keep you ignorant? Few can.

Few are capable of overcoming the human tendency to chase externals and be in a constant state of ignorance. But we should all strive for the truth, the truth of ourselves. It's really hard nonetheless. It requires taking the red pill. It requires that we hurt the Ego. It's a path of winding discomfort and uncertainty. Most people simply don't have what it takes. They might try but invariably fall back into comfort and familiarity, and as a result, they don't grow. They don't become self-actualized. They never live the life they truly deserve.

Only through pain do we grow.

This reminds me of another Arnold quote from Pumping Iron where he says something to the effect of: growth comes past the burn. And he is so right. To pull out results in anything in our lives, we must go *past the burn.* We must go far beyond comfort. We grow through pain, discomfort, and turmoil. It's the yin/yang, positive and negative, night and day, happiness and misery, they all share the same thing: balance of opposing forces.

Inherent in each of us are forces that are always at battle. For us to fully experience happiness we must know what sadness and pain is. The definition of each is how they compare to the opposite. Make sense? We literally need one to have the other. That is what balance is about. For every positive there is a negative lurking around somewhere. Instead of trying to ignore this fact of life, accept it. Then use it to your advantage.

Remind yourself that it's OK to make mistakes; that it's how you learn and become better. Let your Ego experience pain slowly. Take baby steps in challenge it. No one expects you to change your personality over night. That's not practical. But if you can start doing things outside your comfort zone on a regular basis, you will, in time, make real, lasting change. Eventually, you will tame the Ego and become its master. When this happens, you will have attainted true power. The power of yourself.

I wish you the best of luck in this journey. Actually, no. You don't need luck. You need work. Do the work, open your mind, and email me if you need help along the way: ismynamecolin@gmail.com.

Yours in Fitness,

-Colin Stuckert

P.S. If you enjoyed this book please, please leave me a review. This helps me in more ways than one. Thank you so much! Visit www.GymLifeBook.com to leave a review.

P.P.S. Remember: **Train No Matter What**—no excuses. Check out www.GymLifeClub.com to get on my mailing list and get a ton of useful and free content right to your inbox.

P.S.P.S. If you are interested in learning how to cook, check out my second book www.GymLifeCook.com.

Resources

One Page Action Reference Plan
Get the PDF at www.GymLifeClub.com

An easy-to-remember template for your average training week:

Lift weights and train conditioning three times a week.
Do something longer-distance at least once a week.
Do at least one maintenance session a week.
outdoors and do random stuff at least once a week.
Walk every day.

A Hypothetical Training Week:

Monday: Squats followed by a sled-conditioning workout. 15 minutes of skill work at a moderate pace.
Tuesday: Play a pick-up basketball game. A 20-minute walk after dinner. A few sets of push-ups and stretching at home.
Wednesday: Bench press and upper body accessory work. Row 2500m at a slow-med page. Yoga for 15 minutes as a cool-down.
Thursday: Rest. Walk on the beach. Relax and smell the roses. This is known as an "off day."
Friday: Active recovery session and skill work for 1.5 hours in the gym. Legs sore from earlier in week so decide to work upper-body gymnastics (handstands, dips, rings). Ride bike for 20-minutes at a medium pace to speed up recovery.
Saturday: Lifting session of deadlift, Olympic weightlifting work, and GHD sit-ups. Beach volleyball, walk on beach, enjoy a hard-earned cheat meal.
Sunday: Five-mile bike ride at a leisurely pace. Spend two hours prepping food for week. Do 100 push-ups, sit-ups, and squats at home at a slow-to-medium pace.

A Workout:

Body Temp Warm-up: Jog, Row, and move for 5 minutes until you break a sweat.

Dynamic Warm-up: Do movement based exercises at slow/light intensity to warm-up and loosen your joints.

Strength: Perform one or two main lifts a day to failure. Follow a program or stick with 5 sets of 5 at a weight you can barely complete on your last set.

Accessory Exercises: Choose 2-5 complimentary exercises and perform 8-15 reps over 3-5 sets. For example, do pistols (single-leg squats), weighted lunges, glute-ham raises on your squat days and do dips, floor presses and clapping push-ups on your chest/shoulder day.

Conditioning: Complete 5-25 minutes of high-intensity conditioning work.

Cool-down - Stretch, jog, walk, and keep moving for 5 minutes to let your body cool down gradually.

Set Schemes:
10 sets of 2 reps
8 sets of 4 reps
6 sets of 3 reps
5 sets of 5 reps
3 sets of 10
2 sets of 15+
1 set of 21+

Conditioning types:
AMRAP (as many rounds or reps as possible in X time) 5, 7, 9, 10, 12, 15, 20+ minutes
For Time: 2,3,4, 5+ rounds of 2, 3, 4, 5+ exercises for X reps (example= 5 rounds of 10 pull-ups, 10 pushups)
For Time: 100 reps of X
Tabata interval: any exercise or combination of exercises (4 min interval = 20 seconds work, 10 seconds rest until 4 minutes is

complete)
10 50m sprints with rest between

Body Temp warm-ups (3-5 minutes of light activity):
Row 500m
Run 500m
5 minutes jump rope
Incline walks
Bike

Dynamic Stretching Warm-ups (5-7 minutes of movement-based stretching and moving)(mix these up in various reps and sets):
Squats
Lunges
Arm slaps
Arm circles
Wrist rolls
Neck rolls
Side bends
Runner's lunge
Push-ups
Sit-ups
Jumping jacks

Big Lifts for Strength (choose 1-2 for day):
Back Squat and variants: Front Squat, Overhead Squat, Box Squat
Deadlift and variants: sumo, stiff leg, Romanian,
Press and variants: push press, jerk, split jerk, seated
Bench Press and variants: floor press, DB press, incline, decline
Clean and variants: squat, power
Snatch and variants: squat, power

Common accessory exercises (choose 2-4 per strength exercise above as a compliment):
Squats
Deadlifts

Press
Jerk
Push-ups
Dips
Pull-ups
GHD sit-ups
Back extensions
Good mornings
Clean
Snatches
Kettle bell swings

Conditioning (5-20 minutes of various conditioning modalities):
5 mins - 10 mins - 12 mins - 15 mins - 20 mins - 30 mins - 60
minutes (sometimes)
Strongman
Circuits
Intervals (Tabata)
Swimming
Biking
Hiking
Play a sport

Resources:
Home workouts: Trainingbox.tv
The 5/3/1 Program by Jim Wendler
Starting Strength by Mark Rippetoe
GymnasitcsWOD.com
MobilityWOD.com

Home/Travel WOD workouts requiring no equipment:
-For Time: 10 rounds of: 10 push-ups, 10 sit-ups, 10 squats
-For Time: 50 squats, 50 push-ups, 50 sit-ups
-For Time: 5 rounds of: Run 50m, 10 push-ups
-As many rounds as possible in 10 minutes of: 7 squats, 7 push-ups,
15 sit-ups

-Tabata squats - do as many squats as you can for 20 seconds, rest for 10. Repeat for 4 minutes
-For time: Run 1 mile, 100 Pull-ups, 200 Push-ups, 300 Squats, Run 1 mile
-4x 400M sprints - rest between
-10x 50m Sprint
-Run 1/2 mile 50 air squats – 3 rounds.
-10-9-8-7-6-5-4-3-2-1 sets of sit-ups and a 100 meter sprint between each set.
-Three rounds of: Run 800 meters, 50 Supermans, 50 Sit-ups
-10 push-ups, 10 sit ups, 10 squats – 10x rounds
-200 air squats for time
-3 rounds for time of: Sprint 200m, 25 push-ups
-Run 1 mile, lunging 30 steps every 1 minute.
- 30-60 second handstand hold on wall and 20 air squats, 5 rounds.
-100 air squats for time
-100 burpees for time
-50 burpees for time
-For time: 4 rounds of: 10 broad jumps, 10 push ups, 10 sit ups
-10 air squats every 1 minute of your 1 mile run
-Run 1 mile for time